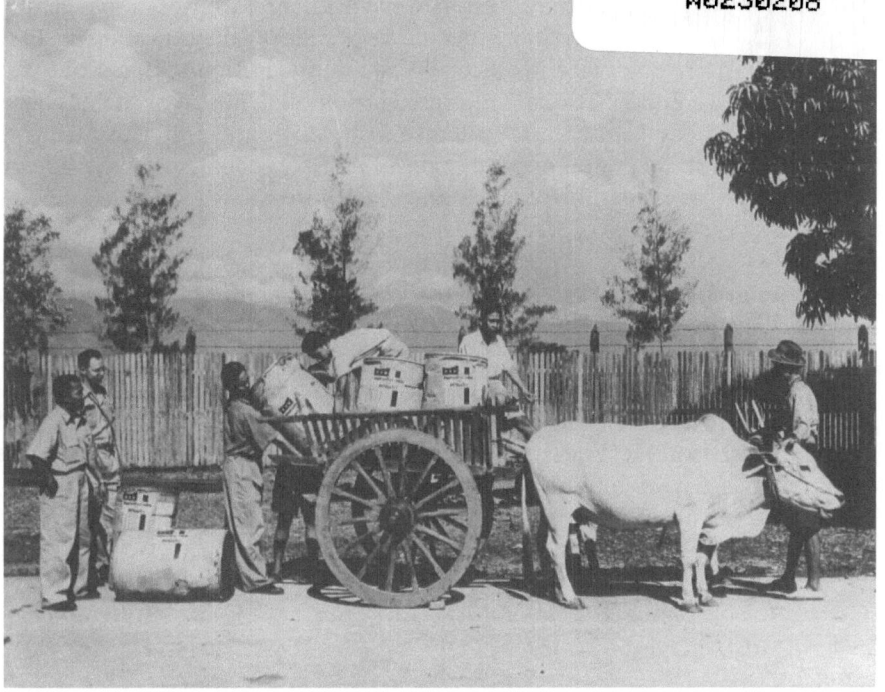

Frontispiece Part of 200 Tons of DDT shipped to Bangkok by ICA, unloaded by ox-carts reach remote inland villages of Thailand. Dr. Term and Thurman closely supervise the work.

An undated ICA photo possibly dating to the late 1950s. Part of 200 tons of DDT shipped to Bangkok by ICA are unloaded on ox carts to reach the remote inland villages of Thailand. Dr. Term and Mr. Thurman closely supervised the work.

Note: The ICA or International Cooperation Administration was a US governmental agency that operated between 1955-61, responsible for foreign assistance and non-military security programs.
Photocredit: ICA USAID Asia
https://www.flickr.com/photos/usaidasia/6006465722/in/album-72157627506230488/

"This book is a welcome addition to the historiography of global health. Its unique focus on region-specific approaches to examining disease eradication allows it to historicise postcolonial nation-states, Cold War politics, and international aid organizations. The range of themes here; from primary health infrastructure in postcolonial India to querying the concept of erosion of civic space in ASEAN countries at the time of coronavirus epidemics, for instance, will interest research scholars as well as the curious general reader."

Nandini Bhattacharya, *Associate Professor (South Asian History and History of Medicine), Department of History, University of Houston*

"This volume pioneers the field with an explicit argument for regional history to fill the gaps between global history and transnational and national history. The studies are comprehensive and informative on major issues of integration and divergence of regional history, illustrated by the policies and politics of public health from the Cold War to the pandemic of Covid-19."

Professor Liping Bu, *Reid Knox Professor and Chair, Alma College, Michigan*

The Geopolitics of Health in South and Southeast Asia

This book analyzes the complexity of South and Southeast Asia in international health, taking into account the impact of the geopolitics of the Cold War on the development of public health and development in the regions.

In light of the recent health pandemic, which has mobilized experts and governments and led to a securitized approach to global health, this book offers a regional approach to global health histories. The chapters provide case studies ranging from the Cold War to the present time and covering countries from across South and Southeast Asia. Contributors analyze issues related to disease control, an adjunct to wider Cold War geopolitics. They also examine the responses of regional organizations, particularly the ASEAN (Association of Southeast Asian Nations) and SAARC (South Asian Association for Regional Cooperation), toward COVID-19. Collectively, the book illustrates how narrowly conceived global health programs implemented by aid agencies failed to account for the local, national or regional contexts.

Situating health in South and Southeast Asia in broader global contexts, the book will be a valuable contribution to the History of Medicine and Health and Political Economy of South and Southeast Asia.

Vivek Neelakantan is a Southeast Asian medical historian and a 2023 Brocher Visiting Fellow, sponsored by the Brocher Foundation, Switzerland. His current research investigates the origins of primary healthcare in Southeast Asia from a transnational perspective.

The Geopolitics of Health in South and Southeast Asia

Perspectives from the Cold War to COVID-19

**Edited by
Vivek Neelakantan**

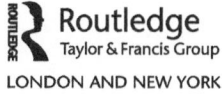

LONDON AND NEW YORK

First published 2023
by Routledge
4 Park Square, Milton Park, Abingdon, Oxon OX14 4RN

and by Routledge
605 Third Avenue, New York, NY 10158

Routledge is an imprint of the Taylor & Francis Group, an informa business

British Library Cataloguing-in-Publication Data
A catalogue record for this book is available from the British Library

Library of Congress Cataloging-in-Publication Data
Names: Neelakantan, Vivek, editor.
Title: The geopolitics of health in South and Southeast Asia : perspectives from the Cold War to COVID-19 / edited by Vivek Neelakantan.
Description: Abingdon, Oxon ; New York, NY : Routledge, 2023. | Series: Routledge contemporary Asia series; 83 | Includes bibliographical references and index.
Identifiers: LCCN 2022041116 (print) | LCCN 2022041117 (ebook) | ISBN 9781032364537 (hardback) | ISBN 9781032364520 (paperback) | ISBN 9781003332060 (ebook)
Subjects: LCSH: Public health--Political aspects--South Asia--History. | Public health--Political aspects--Southeast Asia--History. | Medical policy--South Asia--History. | Medical policy--Southeast Asia--History. | World health--Political aspects--History. | World politics--Health aspects--History. | Public health--International cooperation--History.
Classification: LCC RA541.S64 G46 2023 (print) | LCC RA541.S64 (ebook) | DDC 362.10959--dc23/eng/20221117
LC record available at https://lccn.loc.gov/2022041116
LC ebook record available at https://lccn.loc.gov/2022041117

ISBN: 978-1-032-36453-7 (hbk)
ISBN: 978-1-032-36452-0 (pbk)
ISBN: 978-1-003-33206-0 (ebk)

DOI: 10.4324/9781003332060

Typeset in Times New Roman
by KnowledgeWorks Global Ltd.

Contents

Illustrations

Figures

Map

Tables

Acknowledgments

In the course of writing this volume, I have incurred a trail of intellectual debts. I would like to thank Liping Bu, Reid Knox Chair and Professor of American History at Alma College, Michigan for encouraging me to work on a regional approach to global history in 2021. Over the past decade or so, Liping inspired me and other young historians of my generation to think about the policy ramifications of major landmarks in global history. I would like to dedicate this book to Liping for her tireless dedication in mentoring young historians to realize their true potential.

Preliminary research for the volume was conducted at the Rockefeller Archive Center, New York Public Library, and Tozzer Library at Harvard during the spring of 2019 as a Consortium for the History of Science, Technology and Medicine (CHSTM) Research Fellow from India, sponsored by the Wellcome Trust for the project titled "Southeast Asia and the Beginnings of the Primary Health Paradigm, 1948–78." I am particularly indebted to Lee Hiltzik and the Rockefeller Archive Center archivists for hosting me in 2019 as CHSTM Fellow. The edited volume constitutes a part of a larger project "From Bandoeng to Alma Ata: Southeast Asia and the Beginnings of the Primary Health Paradigm, 1937–78," for which I have been awarded a Brocher Residency (2023). I am particularly indebted to archivists Marie Villemin Partow and Reynald Erard at the WHO headquarters, Geneva for helping me remotely access WHO archival documents during the current COVID crisis (2021–22) that I would not have been able to otherwise access from India.

Contributors to the volume were carefully chosen based on how their abstracts synchronized with the concept nôte. I am thankful to all the contributors for supporting me thick and thin through what was otherwise a difficult year. The biggest challenge I faced along with many contributors was battling COVID-19. I am grateful to Liping Bu and Nandini Bhattacharya for their comments on individual chapters that strengthened the overall quality of the argument. I would like to place on record my indebtedness to Dorothea Schaefter, Saraswathy Narayan, and the Routledge team for being so supportive during the production process.

Note on Thai Patronymics

Thais prefer to be referred to by their first name rather than the patronymic even in academic writing. For example, Sulak Sivaraksa would be referred to as Sulak for the second time in the text.

Contributors

Khoo Ying Hooi is Head and Senior Lecturer at the Department of International and Strategic Studies at the University of Malaya. Her research interests lie at the intersection of human rights, democratization, and civil society actors, focusing on Southeast Asia. Before her academic career, she worked at the Human Rights Commission of Malaysia as the Head of International Issues and Cooperation.

Shirish Kavadi is an independent Medical Historian and a Guest Lecturer at the Symbiosis International University in Pune, India. His research interest includes the history and politics of health and medicine with a focus on medical philanthropy. His ongoing project investigates the Rockefeller Foundation's engagement with medical education and research in post-independent India.

Eva-Maria Knoll is a Senior Researcher at the Institute for Social Anthropology at the Austrian Academy of Sciences. A medical anthropologist by training, her research interests include national and manmade crisis in the Indian Ocean world and the biosocial impact of inherited blood disorders, with special expertise on the Maldives and its history. Since 2013, she serves as a member of the jury that nominates Austria's Best Science Books for the Federal Ministry of Education, Science, and Research.

Vivek Neelakantan is a Southeast Asian medical historian and a 2023 Brocher Visiting Fellow, sponsored by the Brocher Foundation, Switzerland. His monograph *Science, Public Health and Nation-Building in Soekarno-Era Indonesia* examines Indonesia's relations with the WHO during the Cold War and the appropriation of social medicine by nationalist physicians. The monograph has been translated into Bahasa Indonesia. His current research investigates the origins of Primary Healthcare in Southeast Asia from a transnational perspective. He was the 2018–19 Consortium for the History of Science, Technology, and Medicine Research Fellow. His research has been featured in leading international journals including *ISIS Current Bibliography, Wellcome Open Research, Bijdragen tot de Taal-, Land-en Volkenkunde,* and *Southeast Asian Studies.*

Davisakd Puaksom is an Associate Professor in the Department of History at Naresuan University, Thailand. His defining article "Of Germs, Public Hygiene and the Healthy Body: The Making of the Medicalizing State in Thailand," was published in *The Journal of Asian Studies* in 2007. Davisakd has published extensively on medicine, ethnic relations, and the state.

Introduction

Vivek Neelakantan

Contemporary South Asia is at the brink of several conflicts. Insurgency has affected parts of Kashmir, Baluchistan, Assam, and the tribal belt of East central India. Sri Lanka—an island nation in the Indian Ocean that emerged from nearly 25 years of ethnic strife in 2009—is facing political and economic unrest following a default on its external debt that ignited the April 2022 protests. The World Bank- and the IMF-imposed austerity measures to restructure Sri Lanka's ailing economy could probably reverse the country's successes in providing universal healthcare despite limited resources.[1] Nepal has emerged from decades of Maoist insurgency whereas Afghanistan has experienced continual strife since the Soviet invasion in 1979. Between 2017 and 2018, Bangladesh experienced a moderate level of political violence relative to the rest of South and Southeast Asia. These events involved political militias and student wings of the major political parties: the Bangladesh Chhatra League (associated with the ruling party) and Bangladesh Jatiotabadi Chatra Dal (associated with the opposition).[2] Conflict has cost the region dearly. Poor social determinants of health have fueled grassroots rebellion and insurgency in some cases.

South Asia comprises a diverse set of countries ranging from small island states such as the Maldives with a population less than one million to India: soon to replace China as the world's most populous country with an estimated population of approximately 1.4 billion. The South Asian Association for Regional Cooperation (SAARC)—a geopolitical grouping comprising of Bangladesh, Bhutan, The Maldives, Nepal, Pakistan, Sri Lanka, and India, founded in December 1985 as a platform to promote regional collaboration and economic development—suffers from policy paralysis due to bilateral differences between India and Pakistan.

Despite their geographic, socio-linguistic, ethnoreligious, economic, and political differences, all countries of the region face the triple burden of communicable diseases, lifestyle diseases, and a growing recognition of the impact of psychiatric disorders, injuries, and violence. Gender disparities, under-nutrition, and social inequities remain widespread across South Asia and over 300 million people remain in widespread poverty.[3] Zulfiqar Bhutta and Samiran Nundy advocate promoting public health priorities across

DOI: 10.4324/9781003332060-1

South Asia as an important bridge to peace.[4] This in turn, would involve scaling up investments in human development.

Regional cooperation is central to achieving the implementation of the United Nations (UN) 2030 Agenda for Sustainable Development—with 17 Sustainable Development Goals (SDGs) adopted globally in 2015. The SDGs recognize that ending poverty and social deprivation must accompany strategies that improve health and education, reduce social inequality, and boost economic growth. SDG 16 sets targets for peace, justice, and strong institutions and SDG 17 calls for partnerships to attain these goals. South Asian physicians can lead their respective governments in setting up a regional taskforce to monitor progress and support action towards attainment of the SDGs.

The Idea of South/Southeast Asia

South Asia is a neutral term to refer to a geopolitically complex region that is colloquially known as the Indian Subcontinent. The idea of South Asia is interesting for four reasons. First, it refers to a region where the world's major religions associated with different civilizations have been interacting and challenging the notion that a region forms a cultural realm. Second, the ambivalent and contradictory nature of British colonialism, which on the one hand laid the foundations for a mental representation of the region through its unification policies, and on the other hand contributed to divisions between states and across common cultures at the time of independence (1947).[5] Third, the Subcontinent has been characterized by a tragic history that witnessed many partitions, rendering the notions of region and regionalism particularly sensitive.[6] Fourth, the peculiar dominating position of a single country, India, and the specific nature of Pakistan that was established in the name of religion gives region and regionalism a unique flavor as compared to regional constructions in other parts of the world.[7]

The idea of South Asia emerged only by the 1970s and was an imposed one in response to the formation of other comparatively successful regional groupings such as the Association of Southeast Asian Nations (ASEAN, founded 1967). Hostile relations between India and Pakistan have cast a shadow on regional integration from the beginning (both countries have fought three wars). The SAARC—conceived as a mechanism to promote regional integration—has registered sluggish progress since its inception in 1985 as compared to its counterparts such as the ASEAN. Though the region has been experiencing multiple terrorist threats, the SAARC Regional Convention on Suppression of Terrorism signed in Kathmandu in 1987 has been a non-starter.[8] This is so true that for India and a select number of South Asian countries such as Bangladesh, Bhutan, and Nepal, the idea of sub-regional cooperation has emerged as an effective substitute for SAARC.[9]

The India-centeredness of SAARC is obvious. The country accounts for more than two-thirds of South Asia's area, over three-quarters of the region's population, GDP, and military. Every other South Asian state is small in comparison to India. As Ashis Nandy notes, "South Asia is the only region in the world where most states define themselves not by what they are, but by what they are not. Pakistan, Sri Lanka, and Nepal try desperately not to be India; Bangladesh has taken up the more onerous responsibility of avoiding being both India and Pakistan."[10] There is another reason for the Indo-centricity of the SAARC. India's borders (inclusive of maritime borders) touch those of every country of the region excluding Afghanistan. Shared land or maritime borders have resulted in all kinds of bilateral tensions across South Asia, in most of which India is the common factor.

As is the case of South Asia, Southeast Asia is a geopolitical construct. Even today, very few among the region's population—approximately 682 million or 8.58% of the global population of 7.96 billion (according to the July 2022 UN estimate)—consider themselves truly Southeast Asian. The older Chinese notion of *nan-yang* alluded to the southern region to be reached by sea. Its Japanese derivate *nampō* stretched out broadly into what the Americans would later refer to as the Southwest Pacific in official documents. As such, Southeast Asia as a significant political term emerged only by the summer of 1943 with the creation of Lord Mountbatten's Southeast Asia Command, an offshoot of the traditional Indian Command.[11] But the Command was based in Ceylon (known as Sri Lanka since 1972) and included the British Raj's northeastern frontiers (neither in Southeast Asia today) whereas the Dutch East Indies (today known as Indonesia), British Malaya, Singapore, and American Philippines—under Japanese occupation at the time—were excluded from the Command Area due to Japanese assault.[12] The naming of Southeast Asia was a clear response to the historical fact that by 1943, Emperor Hirohito's armies controlled the entire stretch between British Burma and American Philippines. The notion of Southeast Asia gained political currency by the Pacific War (1941–45). Yet, the precise political boundaries of the region remained undefined until the establishment of the ASEAN in 1967.[13]

The ambiguity of defining *what* constituted Southeast Asia could be attributed to four historical factors. First, the region lacked a historic hegemonic power like the Ottomans of the Near East or the Mughals of India. Second, the extraordinary religious diversity of the region —once Islam gained a foothold in the thirteenth century, and Christianity, beginning in the sixteenth century—broke up what was essentially a Hindu-Buddhistic syncretic civilization.[14] Third, the region was imperially fragmented by the nineteenth century with the exception of Siam (Thailand since 1932) that served as a buffer state between British Burma and French Indochina and maintained its political independence. Benedict Anderson notes that unlike Africa, imperialism did not come to Southeast Asia in a late nineteenth-century rush but stretched across centuries. Each European power, jealous of, and rivalrous with its competitors, closed off its colonial possessions from the rest such that at the turn of the twentieth century, young educated people in Batavia (Jakarta) knew more about Amsterdam than they did about Cambodia. Fourth, remote, heterogeneous, and imperially segmented, the region was late in its unitary naming.[15]

The aftermath of the Pacific War and the rapid onset of decolonization coincided with the Cold War and the sustained US attempt to replace Japan with a single regional hegemon. The Southeast Asian Treaty Organization (SEATO) was born in 1954 in Manila in a feat of Cold War gerrymandering.[16] The SEATO's purview was vaguely defined and included the unspecified general area of Southeast Asia, the undefined South Pacific region and a member state Pakistan that had joined the Organization for anti-Indian reasons.[17] The SEATO was beset with contradictions. Whereas on one hand the SEATO endeavored to uphold equal rights and self-determination of peoples, on the other hand the Organization vehemently opposed any attempt to alter the status quo of the territorial integrity and sovereignty of British territories, particularly Singapore, Brunei, and Malaya. Only during the 1960s did the SEATO members—namely Philippines and Thailand—moot the idea of regional integration. In 1961, newly-independent Malaya joined the Philippines and Thailand in forming an Association of Southeast Asia (ASA)—a union that lasted until 1967—when Indonesia and Singapore combined with ASA to constitute the ASEAN.

The ambiguous position of Burma (now known as Myanmar) in South Asia—first, as a province of British India (1824–1937), the subsequent independence from British India in 1935, transfer of power in 1948, and accession to ASEAN in mid-1997—reveal the porosity of the notion of South and Southeast Asia as a region.[18] Unlike the delineation of Southeast Asia by ASEAN, the region of South Asia is not precisely defined in the SAARC Charter. Likewise, Afghanistan could claim SAARC membership but was not among the seven founding members of the geopolitical grouping when it was founded in 1985 due to Soviet occupation of the country. Pakistan initially opposed Afghanistan's SAARC's membership due to the disputed Durand line dividing both neighbors. Yet, Pakistan's support to Afghanistan's SAARC accession in 2007 was conditioned by its strategic partnership with the US.[19] The role of the USA and its policies is also significant in shaping perceptions on Afghanistan's link with South Asia. In the aftermath of the 9/11 terror attacks, Washington coined the AfPak term to achieve political and military objectives by the USA. Afghanistan's SAARC membership poses significant challenges due to the country's position as a war-torn country and its conflictual relationship with Pakistan.

ASEAN: A Microcosm of Global Health

The ASEAN— a region of increasing geopolitical clout, attributed to Asia's global ascent since the 1990s—comprises the states of Brunei, Cambodia, Indonesia, Laos, Malaysia, Myanmar, the Philippines, Singapore, Thailand,

and Vietnam. The region teems with enormous social, ethnic, religious, economic, and political diversity across and within countries. An underlining feature of regional health across the ASEAN is the disparate health status of the population, attributed to rapid but inequitable economic growth. Indonesia is the most populous Southeast Asian nation (276 million) whereas Brunei being the least populous (449,002), according to the World Bank estimates for 2022.[20] Despite a steady improvement of the region's health indicators since the 1950s, continued civil war in Myanmar since the country's independence in 1948 has undermined the country's gains in key health indicators such as life expectancy. For example, Myanmar's average life expectancy for 2020 (67.36 years) is lower than Singapore (83.74), Southeast Asia's best performer.[21] Southeast Asia's peculiar geography has made the region vulnerable to natural disasters such as typhoons, flooding, earthquakes, and environmental pollution. Climate change could exacerbate the spread of infectious diseases.

In 2015, ASEAN leaders identified healthcare as a priority sector that could contribute towards regionwide integration. The ASEAN Free Trade Area intends to augment the region's competitive advantage as a net provider of healthcare services that are oriented towards the world market. From an economic perspective, the opening of healthcare markets promises substantial economic gains. At the same time, however, this process could also intensify existing challenges in promotion of equitable access to healthcare within countries. It could also lead to undesirable outcomes whereby only the better-off will receive benefits from the liberalization of trade policy in health.[22] Furthermore, the export of human resources in health—from comparatively poorer countries of the region to richer countries of the region—has accentuated the shortage of medical personnel, particularly in the former. Rapid economic development and reduction of family size in Singapore and Thailand have motivated both countries to open doors to in-migration of migrant labor from the Philippines, Vietnam, and Indonesia. Migrant workers are unlikely to be enrolled in national health insurance schemes of their host country and may suffer from inadequate access to health services.

Southeast Asia has undergone unprecedented demographic transition in terms of fertility reduction, population aging, and rural-to-urban migration. Furthermore, the region also has undergone epidemiological transition, with the disease burden shifting from infectious diseases to chronic conditions. Rapid urbanization, population movements, high-density living, environmental changes such as agriculture and livestock intensification, deforestation, and climate change have raised concerns about Emerging Infectious Diseases in the region, but these outbreaks have provided the impetus for regional cooperation.[23] Outbreaks of Severe Acute Respiratory Syndrome (SARS) and H5N1 Avian Influenza across much of the region in 2003 have attracted international attention toward Southeast Asia. Despite the region's centrality with respect to Emerging Infectious

Diseases, frailties and differences in surveillance systems across ASEAN states hamper timely reporting of these diseases.[24] Emerging Infectious Diseases have the potential to upend the region's economy. For example, the estimated cost of SARS to the economies of East Asia and the ASEAN was $18 billion that worked out to US$2 million per person infected.[25] The Avian Influenza outbreak led to a 93% decline in poultry meat exports from Thailand between 2003 and 2004 and led to a culling of 45 million birds in Vietnam at an estimated cost of $118 million.[26]

The Avian Influenza outbreak served as a catalyst to ASEAN members to strengthen disease surveillance that included integrating elements of animal health, the deployment of rapid response teams to track outbreaks, and the building of biosafety level 3 laboratories for virus sequencing. ASEAN member states have endorsed a regional mechanism on animal health and zoonoses. The integration of animal and human health has been at the center of WHO's Asia-Pacific Strategy on Emerging Diseases (APSED)—an ambitious strategic framework that aims to develop mechanisms for information sharing between the animal and human health sectors both at regional and country levels, in partnership with the Food and Agriculture Organization and the World Organization for Animal Health.[27] Thriving private healthcare in many countries increasingly poses challenges to disease surveillance. Similar challenges arise from decentralized health systems—for example, in Indonesia and the Philippines, where local health authorities have become less active in case reporting compared with other countries. Where vertical disease-specific surveillance programs have been developed, such as in Cambodia, there is a risk that parallel surveillance and laboratory testing systems—especially those funded through overseas aid related to pandemic influenza preparedness—draw on limited existing capacity and contribute to a duplication of efforts.[28]

International and regional collaboration related to sharing of viral samples in the region have been impeded by underlying national anxieties of ASEAN member states related to the patenting of vaccines and pharmaceuticals by multinational drug companies. The patented products are sold at high prices that in turn, disproportionately benefit high-income countries. In February 2007, amidst a global concern about the threat of pandemic influenza, Indonesia's health Minister Siti Fadilah Supari announced that her country would no longer share Avian Influenza virus samples with the WHO. She contended that her country had "viral sovereignty."[29] Supari pressed the WHO to accept the idea that the nation, not the world community as represented by the WHO, held the rights to viral samples. She argued that the 1992 UN Convention on Biological Diversity, which protects a nation's rights to the genetic diversity found within its borders, extends even to the microbial diversity found in Indonesia and obviates Indonesia's obligations under the international sample-sharing mechanism of the WHO. Thus, Indonesia's minister of health demanded the international community recognize that the viral material underlying the international influenza regime was the property of Indonesia, required the consent of the Indonesian government to be shared, and needed a formal Material Transfer Agreement to move between countries.[30] A dispute over property rights between the Indonesian government and an Australian pharmaceutical company that used H5N1 viral strains sourced from Indonesia to produce and market the H5N1 vaccine triggered Supari's controversial decision.

To reinforce Supari's notion of "viral sovereignty," Indonesia held a high-level meeting that included national health ministers and the WHO officials in 2007. Delegates discussed how samples could be shared equitably and fairly. They adopted the "Jakarta Declaration," a document that emphasized sharing benefits (including epidemiological data and affordable vaccines) resulting from the circulation of biological specimens. Supari's stance brought to light the need for an expanded sense of materiality in response to the virus: curing ill patients would not only require cladistics and viral sequencing but also drug distribution across the Indonesian archipelago and the means to acquire them.[31] Supari feared that although the seed stock for the H5N1 Avian Influenza may come from Indonesia, developed countries would have full control over the production and distribution of vaccine stocks and determine which countries could access them.[32] In 2008, after a protracted negotiation with the WHO, Indonesia finally agreed to share H5N1 Avian Influenza sequences but not the viral samples. In 2009, the country refused to share virus samples with the Global Influenza Surveillance Network as initial efforts to create a more equitable framework for the purchase and distribution of vaccines did not lead to substantial results due to disagreements between Indonesia and high-income nations. The latter were reluctant to accept Indonesia's and Thailand's suggestion of legally-binding obligations to share the benefits of vaccines that accrued from the sharing of biological samples.[33]

The implementation of the program for the control of Emerging Infectious Diseases in Southeast Asia is contingent on the support of international aid agencies such as the Asian Development Bank, the World Bank, or the Rockefeller Foundation. Overseas development assistance in health highlights priorities of international aid agencies and mainstream global health such as HIV/AIDS prevention whereas endemic diseases such as yaws afflicting individual countries are neglected. Furthermore, bilateral tensions such as the Thai-Cambodian dispute centered on the Preah Vihear Temple, the re-imposition of military rule in Myanmar (2021), or ongoing conflicts such as the insurgency in southern Thailand since 1948 could stymie regional health initiatives.

Since 1948, the WHO disembarked on a program of regionalization. The proposed regional office for Southeast Asia was partitioned into the WHO Regional Office for Southeast Asia (SEARO) and the Western Pacific (WPRO) on geopolitical lines that were not precisely delineated. In turn, the WHO's partitioning of Southeast Asia has impeded regional collaboration related to the collection of epidemiological data. Nonetheless, a 1999

Rockefeller Foundation-funded transnational initiative, the Mekong Basin Disease Surveillance—inclusive of Myanmar, China's Yunnan province and Guangxi Zhuang Autonomous Region, Vietnam, Cambodia, Laos, and Thailand—straddle both the SEARO and WPRO member states. For example, in 1999, there was a serious outbreak of cholera in a remote northern province of Cambodia on the Vietnam border. Cambodia recognized that not only did it need to strengthen community-based surveillance, but also that it could better contain such epidemics if Cambodian and Vietnamese epidemiologists and officials worked together.[34] Since 2007, the scope of the Mekong Basin Disease Surveillance has extended beyond disease surveillance. For instance, Thailand dispatched cross-border medical aid to Myanmar after cyclone Nargis in 2008. The completion of a regional tabletop pandemic preparedness exercise in Siem Reap, Cambodia (2007) further serves as an example of transnational collaboration through the initiative.[35]

A Regional Approach to Global Health History

The idea for the edited volume arose from a larger research project, straddling the colonial and postcolonial divide, entitled "From Bandoeng to Alma Ata: Southeast Asia and the Emergence of Primary Health Paradigm, 1937-78." Preliminary data collection for the project—between April and June 2019 at the Rockefeller Archive Center, Tozzer and Schlesinger Libraries (Harvard University), and the New York Public Library— was supported by the Consortium for the History of Science, Technology and Medicine Research Fellowship. Almost a year later, with the onset of the COVID-19 pandemic in 2020, India sought to market itself as the "pharmacy of the world" and supplied medical kits, personal protective equipment, gloves, and essential medicines to its South Asian neighbors as a part of its "Neighborhood First" strategy. The COVID-19 crisis provided India the opportunity to disentangle itself from bilateral disputes with Pakistan and instead, compete with China for regional hegemony in South Asia. The pandemic highlighted that disease control has become an adjunct to geopolitics.

Contributors to the volume include an eclectic mix of medical historians, a medical anthropologist, and an international relations expert, drawn from four nations and two continents. Constituent chapters not only critically examine medical developments across South and Southeast Asia between the Cold War and COVID-19 (1948–2021) but also firmly situate the history of health of individual nations within the broader domain of global health. Drawing on a wide variety of archival sources, oral history interviews, and international relations theory, the contributors collectively investigate the regional history of health and the extent to which the campaign against disease contributed toward regional integration in South and Southeast Asia. The volume will offer a unique perspective that contributed to the formation of a South and Southeast Asian regional identity.

The purpose of the edited volume is to write a regional history of health in South and Southeast Asia from a transnational and comparative perspective located within the shifting context of the Cold War and the rise of China as a hegemonic power in Asia during the era of COVID-19. A regional approach to global health history would trace both international influences and local specificities. Research for the volume revolves around four major cores: (a) the global vectors of disease and the transmission of technical assistance through international aid agencies such as the WHO, as reflected in Chapters 1 and 3; (b) how international organizations affected the region and were in turn, affected by it, a theme broached by Chapters 1 and 3; (c) the regional flow of health challenges, proposed solutions, and the formation of regional epistemic communities particularly the WHO Regional Office for Southeast Asia (SEARO), SAARC, and ASEAN, explored in Chapters 1, 5, and 6; and (d) the influence of the Cold War on the national politics of health, examined in Chapters 1, 2, and 4.

The overarching argument underpinning the volume is that if medical historians of South and Southeast Asian Studies have forsaken region in favor of the nation state, historians of global health have overlooked region in favor of the globe. What is needed in medical history is a regional perspective that would help elucidate how international aid agencies tailored health policies to suit local conditions in ways that were mediated by Cold War and national reconstruction in the post-World War II era.

The post-World War II world order (1945–90) was marked by the onset of the Cold War: military and ideological rivalries between the US and the Soviet Union. The Cold War manifested new forms of conflict and collaboration in international health. Cold War medicine is reflected in two kinds of historical writing. Whereas medical historians tend to focus largely on the institutional histories of the WHO—and to a lesser extent on historical biographies—historians specializing on the Cold War center their narratives on decolonization, nationalism, and socialist internationalism.[36]

In recent syntheses, historians Marcos Cueto, Theodore Brown, and Elizabeth Fee portray the establishment of the WHO in 1948 as the endorsement of the technocratic and biomedical perspective. For example, the widespread application of insecticide DDT to eradicate malaria.[37] Attempts at eradicating malaria and the subsequent failures by 1969 reflected limitations of the American-led industrial vision of modernity based on the assumption that underdeveloped countries would become developed by achieving high levels of industrialization and urbanization, technicalization of agriculture, rapid growth of material production and living standards, and the widespread adoption of modern education and cultural values.[38] Malaria eradication in developing countries ignored the cyclical relationship between disease and poverty while reinforcing the proverbial magic bullet.[39]

Recently, historians have examined the campaigns against malaria and smallpox within the larger context of the Cold War. Elizabeth Fee, Theodore Brown, and Marcos Cueto note that between 1948 and 1956—as the USSR withdrew its membership from the WHO, citing ideological differences with the US—the agency became captive of American geopolitical interests and pursued a narrow program of disease eradication.[40] During the Eisenhower administration, as tensions with the USSR increased, the US Congress made DDT-driven malaria eradication as a part of America's soft-power campaign. In his State of the Union Address (1958), President Eisenhower exhorted the Soviets to join the global eradication of malaria. On the contrary, the USSR called for a new global program against smallpox that competed with the WHO's malaria eradication program.[41] Erez Manela depicts the global smallpox eradication campaign as a striking example of a Cold War paradox, as growing superpower interest in the third world, interest that was born of Cold War competition, helped produced what was arguably the single most successful instance of superpower collaboration in Cold War history. Factors that contributed to the success of the smallpox eradication program included the coupling of US funds with the USSR's vaccine production capacity.[42]

Although global health is read as synonymous with the WHO, it also existed outside the organization's auspices.[43] Dora Vargha examines Hungary, Czechoslovakia, and Poland's experiences with the polio vaccine during the 1950s. The West, while not endorsing the Communist regimes, agreed to provide live poliovirus vaccines. Czechoslovakia, Hungary, and Poland became pioneers in introducing, testing, and applying live poliovirus vaccines. From a broader geopolitical perspective, polio raised uncomfortable questions about the positive side of Communist regimes (i.e., effective epidemic control) and in a short time came to symbolize "neutral" science that broke the barriers between East and West.[44] The centralized organization of polio vaccine trial and immunization in Hungary of the 1950s—which was at the time seen as particularly East European and Communist—later became a model for the WHO's global polio eradication initiative.

During its first decade (1948–58), apart from the Cold War, the WHO had to contend with decolonization and the dissolution of colonial empires as it disembarked on a program of regionalization or decentralizing administrative functions to its regional offices.[45] Three historical studies— that point to the WHO's involvement in decolonization— gave the organization an ambiguous position in international politics. First, during the 1950s, although Portugal was a founder-member of the WHO, the country was locked in Cold War and rising international tensions on one hand while holding on to its colonial possessions on the other. The country tended to walk a political tightrope between constructive engagement and national and international sovereignty.[46] Second, Portuguese Goa's SEARO membership was one of the tools to reinforce Portugal's self-representation as an intercontinental nation-state within decolonizing Southeast Asia and in direct confrontation with the postcolonial nation state, India.[47] Third, (in the context of Africa) concomitant with the WHO's regionalization program (beginning 1948), the future WHO African regional office (AFRO) faced challenges from a parallel regional body: the Commission for Technical Cooperation in Africa to the South of the Sahara (CTCA). The CTCA was a post-World War II Anglo-French initiative that facilitated technical cooperation between African colonies. French administrators had delayed the creation of the AFRO as they feared the regional organization would erode colonial hegemony.[48]

The role of regional health organizations in global health histories has received scant historical attention. Extant scholarship focuses on the ways in which the regional office served as a "contact zone"—the outcome of a product of diplomatic negotiations and shifting combinations of national, colonial, post-colonial, regional, and international interests.[49] Likewise, in the context of smallpox eradication, Sanjoy Bhattacharya highlights the ways in which regional offices interpreted epidemiological guidelines from the WHO Headquarters based on their own understandings of local requirements. These features of "locality" were presented as challenging and inconstant, which meant that program implementation would require frequent re-jigging as political arrangements with different national governments were set up, reconfigured or abandoned.[50] Politics and divergences between WHO and the regional offices overshadowed discussion on health at the SEARO level.

In *Decolonizing International Health: India and Southeast Asia*, Sunil Amrith observes that during the 1950s, the WHO activities across Asia resembled a network with a number of nodal points (projects) between which experts, supplies, and fleets of vans moved constantly. By the mid-1950s, on the eve of the malaria eradication campaign, the organization was responsible for eight projects in Afghanistan; 10 in Burma; 11 in Ceylon; 15 in India; 10 in Indonesia, and 9 in Thailand. The projects encompassed everything from malaria control and demonstration projects using DDT to pilot projects in nursing education and the establishment of statistical infrastructures. Despite their very limited number and localized nature, such projects succeeded in orienting health policy in the region by focusing on specific diseases and campaigns of treatment. There was a remarkable similarity in the health policies adopted by polities as different as those of India, Indonesia, and Burma, each framed within a broader "Southeast Asian" approach to health.[51] Amrith's "Southeast Asian approach to health" does not critically interrogate the influence of the Cold War, the Asian-African Conference, Bandung (1955), and the resultant Communiqué that contributed to the evolution of the "Southeast Asian" approach to health that in turn, influenced the regional character of the SEARO.[52]

Historians have characterized the Asian-African Conference at Bandung variously as: a theatrical performance staged before the world; the zeitgeist of the postcolonial moment; and, the converging forces of decolonization and the Cold War.[53] The Communiqué articulated a collective project against colonialism and imperialism for self-determination and racial-equality, while laying the foundations for the idea of strategic non-alignment in the context of the Cold War.[54] The "Bandung Spirit" underlined the political project of "Third Worldism" and the call for a new international economic order by the 1970s.[55] The Communiqué indicated that Bandung participants agreed to provide technical assistance to one another, to the maximum extent practicable, in the form of experts, trainees, pilot projects, and equipment for demonstration purposes; exchange of know-how and establishment of national, and where possible, regional training and research institutes for imparting technical knowledge and skills in cooperation with the existing international agencies. Yet, health was not explicitly mentioned in the Communiqué.[56]

Subsequent to the Sino-Soviet split of the late 1950s, China used medical diplomacy to counter the American and Soviet influence in non-aligned nations. Jeremy Youde notes that by the early 1970s—as China exported the so-called barefoot doctor model to Africa—medical teams focused less on emergency care and more instead on bringing preventative health to rural areas of the continent.[57] In contrast, the centralized Soviet model of healthcare was perceived as less effective. At the UN, China's increasing medical humanitarian activities helped the country score diplomatic points against Taiwan for the permanent Chinese seat at the Security Council in 1971. Subsequent to its reentry into the WHO in 1973, China used the World Health Assembly (WHA) Meetings to promote its new Third World policy and combat the USSR. Zhou Xun contends that China's rural health delivery system—the Barefoot Doctor program—which involved training program for grassroots health workers and mobilization of health services, linked with mass political campaigns, soon became the inspiration for the Primary Healthcare (PHC) Movement.[58]

Historians have identified at least four factors that contributed to the evolution of PHC Movement. First, the Movement developed in response to the failure of the global malaria eradication campaign. The failure of the malaria eradication program in turn, left the door open for the Soviets to take a leading position in the development of health services. Having fought the battle against the WHO's vertical campaigns of the 1960s, the Soviets sought to gain as much political advantage as possible from what they had accomplished in this field. Their first step was to introduce a draft resolution to the 1970 World Health Assembly on the subject.[59] Second, Kenneth Newell, a WHO staff member who had worked in Indonesia, had become familiar with experiences of medical auxiliaries and was of the conviction that improved food security in rural areas would result in a decrease in infant mortality.[60] Third, the Christian Medical Commission (CMC)—a specialized organization of the World Council of Churches and established in 1968 by medical missionaries working in developing countries—emphasized training of health workers at the grassroots level. In 1970, the CMC financially supported the Jamkhed project in Western India— led by a husband-wife medical team, Rajanikant and Mabelle Arole. Their project aimed to establish an effective health system that involved the community.[61]

Fourth, Newell's advocacy of China's Barefoot Model was supported by the then WHO Director General Halfdan Mahler (1973–88) who was the moving force for the proposed "Health for All."

There is consensus amidst historians that western nations accepted Mahler's idea of universal PHC. On the contrary, the USSR was still in favor of centralized healthcare and condemned the PHC as a retrogressive step. From their perspective, the notion of PHC implied a victory for China and the developing world. This in turn, would undermine the USSR's claim as the people's health provider.[62] When the Chinese delegation to the WHO pressed hard to host the Conference on Primary Healthcare, the USSR began to lobby hard to host the Conference.[63] Alma Ata became the venue for the Conference on PHC (1978) because it was the showcase of achievement for the Soviets in providing centralized healthcare for the remote Kazakhs.[64]

At the Alma Ata Conference, Cold War misunderstandings prevented the Soviets from acknowledging the disconnect between different understandings of PHC.[65] Newell and other Western proponents of PHC noted the lack of community participation in the Soviet health system. Anne-Emanuelle Birn and Nikolai Krementsov note that at the Conference, the Soviets missed an opportunity to showcase their free universal health coverage due to two reasons: (a) the Soviets were of the conviction that the social dimensions of health were self-evident due to the results of the socialist system; and, (b) muted USSR interest in the Conference due to the marginality of the WHO in their health diplomacy since 1948.[66]

After Alma Ata, the WHO almost completely backtracked on its commitment to PHC and instead, adopted a more modest formulation known as Selective Primary Healthcare (SPHC) that the then UNICEF Director James Grant advocated. SPHC meant a package of low-cost technical interventions to tackle the problems of poor countries.[67] SPHC was associated with a set of specific, low-cost interventions captured by the acronym GOBI, derived from the four chief interventions: Growth monitoring to overcome subnormal growth because of inadequate nutrition (an intervention that meant the use of child growth charts by mothers in their homes), Oral rehydration techniques for diarrheal diseases, Breastfeeding, and Immunization. These four interventions seemed easy to monitor and evaluate, and funding appeared easier to obtain because indicators of success could be produced rapidly.[68] A debate developed between advocates of PHC and the supporters of SPHC.

Advocates of PHC criticized the notion of SPHC on the following grounds: (a) SPHC evaluated the costs and benefits of disease within an economic framework; (b) undermined the social causes of disease; (c) relied on structures of dominance, particularly the police and military authorities for implementing nationwide immunization; (d) depended on electronic media for promotion of health campaigns; and, (e) provided an excuse for the state and international agencies to cut back on social expenditure.[69]

On the contrary, proponents of SPHC leveled the following criticisms against PHC: (a) PHC ignored the consideration that good health was contingent on overall economic development rather than the health sector; (b) looked at traditional medicine alternatives as ways of letting the state off the hook, by providing a shabby alternative to the equitable redistribution of healthcare resources; and, (c) enthusiastically advocated community participation as the path to PHC while failing to address the role of the state.[70] US aid agencies, the World Bank, and UNICEF began to prioritize some aspects of GOBI, such as immunization and oral rehydration. They believed that it was a grave error to promote something akin to revolution in developing countries but also naïve to expect changes from their inflexible bureaucracies.[71] As a result, increasing acrimony developed between the PHC-supporting WHO and the SPHC-supporting UNICEF by the early-1980s.

Beginning mid-1980s—with the warming up of the US-Soviet relations following economic crisis and disintegration of the latter—international health was no longer undergirded by Cold War tensions. Anne-Emanuelle Birn contends that if the 1970s witnessed an ascendant role for non-aligned nations at Alma Ata, by the mid-1980s, the interests of the Third World were displaced by the private sector involvement in public health.[72] Since the late-1980s, the business-style orientation of the private sector emphasized success in reaching concrete goals in the improvement of health indicators through management-style performance accountability measures. On the contrary, during the 1970s, health was broadly defined by the Alma Ata Declaration "as a state of complete physical, mental, and social well-being, and not merely the absence of disease or infirmity." Following trenchant criticisms of its inefficient bureaucratic procedures (1990s), the WHO has sought to reinvent itself by adhering to the World Bank's prescription of "investing in health," that sought to emphasize cost effectiveness of specific health interventions.[73]

Since 2000, the World Bank and the WHO have emphasized a Private-Public Partnerships (PPP) model for effective healthcare delivery. The largest PPP, the Global Fund to Fight AIDS, TB and Malaria (established in 2002) as an independent financing entity, disburses grants to developing nations which need to propose concrete short-term fixes to each disease rather than address the underlying social determinants of health.[74]

Contemporary health issues such as HIV/AIDS or SARS have received considerable historical attention in the context of nation-states or cities, although only a few scholars offer a truly regional perspective.[75] A regional perspective is necessary to understand not only the causes of the pandemics but also their legacy—such as the challenges encountered by developing countries in securing access to generic drugs.

Summary of Chapters

The volume seeks to inspire social scientists and health professionals alike to examine global health from a regional perspective. To understand the pervasive role of technical assistance—from the birth of the SEARO, India's quest for pharmaceutical self-sufficiency through a policy of non-alignment, to malaria eradication in Sri Lanka and the Maldives—we must examine external influences such as the Cold War from numerous perspectives and scales. Although the history of regional health transcends the Cold War, in some ways the Cold War is a central aspect to contemporary South and Southeast Asian histories. The legacy of the Cold War in South and Southeast Asia's public health was conspicuous in the emphasis accorded to disease control by the US during the 1950s and 1960s as a means to subvert the growth of communist ideology. Likewise, in the current COVID-19 crisis, India, Japan, Australia, and the US are collaborating in the production and distribution of vaccines to the region—through the Quad alliance—to countervail China's vaccine diplomacy in India's neighborhood. The first four chapters analyze the appropriation and transformation of international aid in South and Southeast Asia during the Cold War era (1945–90) whereas the last two discuss the strengths and the weaknesses of a regional approach to global health in the context of the COVID-19 pandemic.

In Chapter 1, Vivek Neelakantan investigates the establishment of the SEARO in 1948, headquartered at New Delhi, India—the first among six WHO regional offices established between 1948 and 1951 as a part of the Organization's administrative decentralization—in the wider context of the Cold War. Between 1948 and 1956, the USSR and its allies withdrew from the Organization citing ideological differences with the US over socialized medicine whereas the US contended that poverty was the breeding ground of communism. Since disease led to poverty, the US contended that eradicating disease would thwart the spread of communism to newly-independent countries of Asia and Africa. The WHO became captive of US geopolitical interests (1950s) and embarked on a narrow program of disease eradication, a trend also visible in the implementation of the SEARO's campaigns against endemic diseases. Neelakantan notes that during the 1950s, the SEARO's regional agenda consisted of aggregation of member states' requests for technical assistance. During the 1950s, due to Cold War exigencies, as Western aid to Southeast Asia was greater than UN technical assistance, donors would not consult with the WHO or other UN agencies, leading to lopsided developmental assistance that did not reflect local needs. In such situations, the SEARO would assist with priority setting in health and would steer health ministries of member states in the direction of what was reasonably achievable instead of what was desirable. Between 1955 and 1960 at the annual SEARO meetings, Indian, Burmese, and Indonesian leaders alluded to the proverbial Bandung Spirit arising from the Communiqué of the Asian-African Conference at Bandung (1955). The Bandung Spirit emphasized self-sufficiency in economic affairs, solidarity with newly-decolonized nations, and raising peoples' living standards. Yet, it is unclear to what extent the Bandung Spirit influenced the regional character of the SEARO. Third World solidarity in Southeast Asia began to fragment by the mid-1960s due to domestic political factors. For example, the end of the Soekarno-Era of Indonesian politics was precipitated by the September 30, 1965 movement that led to Indonesia's abandonment of the Bandung Spirit and the resultant pull of the country into the Western orbit.

Shirish Kavadi examines various attempts to reform public health in India (1947–57) in the larger Cold War context. Between 1947 and 1957, India's First Minister of Health Rajkumari Amrit Kaur established close working relations with the US, the Rockefeller Foundation, and the WHO to maximize technical assistance for public health. Amrit Kaur sought to locate her own medical projects such as the All India Institute of Medical Sciences (AIIMS) and the Indian Council of Medical Research—modeled on the lines of the Johns Hopkins Medical School—within Nehruvian science, an institution-building project. Kavadi observes that Amrit Kaur's missionary zeal was constrained by the wider Nehruvian commitment towards industrialization and centralized planning that reduced annual budgetary allocations for public health and Prime Minister Jawaharlal Nehru's own reservations about American aid. On the contrary, between 1948 and 1956— as the Soviets had withdrawn their membership from the WHO—they did not participate in the development of India's medical education. But Indo-Soviet relations warmed with the death of Stalin as Nikita Khrushchev's policy of internationalization was inclusive of non-communist states in the aftermath of the Asian-African Conference at Bandung (1955). At the time, Soviet technical assistance in health was only incidental, and instead focused on building India's capacity in the production of organic chemicals and pharmaceutical intermediaries. India's Second Five-Year Plan (1956–61) envisioned a niche for the private sector in the development of the country's pharmaceutical sector. But Nehru was fearful of the monopoly wielded by transnational corporations. Although Santok Singh Sokhey—who served as WHO's Assistant Director of Health Services between 1949 and 1952—brokered Soviet assistance for the establishment of Indian Drugs and Pharmaceuticals Limited (a public sector company), Nehru was equally skeptical about continued technological dependency on the USSR. In Chapter 2, Kavadi argues that India was successful in building state capacity in the production of pharmaceuticals with Soviet aid and Western technological knowhow. The country succeeded in reducing the price of pharmaceuticals by 1970 through a policy of non-alignment that sought to balance between economic self-sufficiency and increased openness to overseas technical assistance. Yet, very little of the notion of economic self-sufficiency articulated in the Bandung Communiqué was ever agreed on a multilateral basis or implemented by the Non-Aligned group.

Eva-Maria Knoll's chapter portrays divergent trajectories of malaria eradication in the Maldives and Sri Lanka, two island states of South Asia, within the broader context of decolonization in the Indian Ocean that coincided with the onset of Cold War tensions. Knoll contends that although malaria eradication arrived comparatively late in the Maldives (around 1965)—at a time when the malaria eradication campaign in SEARO member states was faltering—the island nation successfully eliminated malaria unlike neighboring Sri Lanka. Although the malaria eradication program in Maldives was constrained by weak health infrastructure and a sparse population dispersed across atolls, factors contributing to the elimination of the disease included small island settings that were congenial to quarantine and isolation of infectious cases. On the contrary, given Ceylon's centrality as a plantation economy, the British introduced malaria control measures as early as 1911, insecticide DDT was introduced as a quick fix to the disease by 1947, and by 1963, malaria was virtually eliminated in the island nation. In the nationalist trope of Sinhala leaders, malaria eradication was portrayed as the means to recolonize the Dry Zone of the island nation and restore the ancient glory of the hydraulic civilization of the Sinhala-Buddhist majority. Yet, state-sponsored colonization of the dry zone and irrigation schemes and resistance of the anopheline species to insecticide DDT contributed to the recrudescence of malaria in Sri Lanka between 1967 and 1984. Sri Lanka conforms with mainstream global health history narrative on the origins, rise, and setback of the global malaria eradication program.[76] On the contrary, despite a pronounced febrile history, the Maldives were neglected in British colonial medical interventions and were left behind when the SEARO commenced the malaria eradication campaign by 1957. Maldives' delayed decolonization, negligible caseload, and presumed immunity of the local population to malaria contributed to elimination of the disease. Malaria eradication in the Maldives does not conform to the dominant historiographical narrative on the origins, rise, and setback of the global malaria eradication program. Knoll portrays malaria eradication in the Maldives as a case of successful localization of an international health initiative.

Davisakd Puaksom investigates the local origins of the global movement towards PHC in the context of the activities of the Rural Doctor Society of Thailand since its first abortive inception (1976), its rebirth following the political upheaval of 1978, and the articulation of a rural healthcare agenda. Thai practitioners' vision for rural healthcare was reflected in medical periodicals such as *Warasan sahaphan phaet chonnabot* (*Journal of the Rural Doctor Federation*, 1976) and *Warasan chomrom phaetchonnabot* (Journal *of the Rural Doctor Society*, 1978). The imprint of the Rural Doctor Society was reflected in Thailand's road toward universal healthcare by the early 2000s and the country's resilience during the COVID-19 crisis. In January 2020, the Thai Ministry of Health dismissed the seriousness of the coronavirus crisis whereas by March 2020 the Ministry backpedaled on its earlier decision and imposed a nationwide lockdown that resulted in an exodus of migrant workers from Bangkok to rural areas. Despite stopgap relief measures, Thailand was ranked sixth on the Global Health Security Index. Davisakd credits the relative resilience of the Thai health system to the introduction of Community Health Workers (CHWs) in 1977, partly in response to demands from the Rural Doctor Society. During the exodus of migrant workers to rural areas, CHWs played a pivotal role in educating migrant workers and their families about the infectiousness of COVID, and assisted with contact-tracing.

In Chapter 5, Khoo Ying Hooi analyzes disparate responses to COVID-19 in 2020 across five ASEAN states namely Brunei, Indonesia, Malaysia, the Philippines, and Singapore, that collectively constitute maritime Southeast Asia. Whereas Indonesia adopted less-restrictive social restriction measures instead of a nationwide lockdown, Malaysia issued a Movement Control Order whilst the Philippines implemented a nationwide lockdown. The common denominator underlying COVID control across the five countries under study included elements of securitization that impacted the enjoyment of individual rights. Early ASEAN response to COVID-19 was swift. On January 4, 2020—soon after the regional grouping received notification of unexplained pneumonia-like clusters from Wuhan—the ASEAN Emergency Operations Center was activated to provide situational updates. The ASEAN Secretariat Socio-Cultural Community Department partnered with the Asia Foundation, the Rockefeller Foundation, and the Australian government to assess impact of the pandemic on livelihoods of the poor. Yet, there was a lack of coordination between ASEAN member states to address health issues of migrant workers. ASEAN's multilateral response to the pandemic has been circumscribed by its efforts to promote regional integration rather than a supranational union among members, where individual states cede aspects of sovereignty to the regional grouping.

As the case of ASEAN, the SAARC response to COVID-19 in 2020 was incoherent. Neelakantan observes that India and Bangladesh opted for nationwide lockdowns that were subsequently followed by efforts to scale up social security whilst Pakistan instituted a program of Emergency Cash Transfer to vulnerable groups to mitigate the economic fallout of the pandemic. During the first wave of the pandemic, India convened a meeting of SAARC leaders and instituted the SAARC COVID-19 Emergency Fund. But administration of the Fund suffered from policy paralysis due to bilateral differences between India and Pakistan as the latter viewed the SAARC COVID-19 Emergency Fund as yet another India-led initiative. There was negligible collaboration within SAARC member states on COVID-19 surveillance, or identification of variants. Likewise, as India's vaccine diplomacy sought to counter China's growing influence in South Asia, Pakistan was apparently excluded from the initiative. Neelakantan argues that the capacity of SAARC to mount a regional response to the coronavirus crisis was contingent on the development of national and regional diagnostic capacities and securing timely access to medical supplies and vaccines. Between March 2020 and March 2021—until the onset of the second wave of the pandemic across South Asia—India was partly successful in scaling up its capacity in the manufacture of personal protective equipment and oximeters. Yet, at the onset of the second wave, most SAARC members imported medical supplies from overseas that could have otherwise been sourced from the region at a fraction of the cost. The COVID crisis revealed the underlying weaknesses of South Asian regionalism.

Conclusion: So Why Does a Regional Approach to Global Health Matter?

The COVID-19 pandemic across South and Southeast Asia not only accelerated but also put a brake on regional integration. Diversity of geography, history, and political systems have affected health outcomes across and within countries of both regions. Across South and Southeast Asia, demographic transition is taking place at among the fastest rates compared with other regions of the world in terms of fertility reductions, population aging, and a shift in disease burden from infectious to lifestyle diseases. Migration from rural to urban areas, high-density living in urban conurbations, and climate change provide the perfect recipe for natural disasters and outbreaks of emerging infectious diseases across both regions. Although the coronavirus crisis stimulated regional cooperation across South and Southeast Asia, the difference between ASEAN and SAARC is one of kind rather than degree.

ASEAN's prior experience with SARS and H5N1 Avian Influenza provided an impetus for member states to institutionalize pandemic preparedness and response. When the news of the Wuhan viral outbreak emerged on January 4, 2020, the regional grouping activated its Emergency Operations Center that serves as a surveillance mechanism. Furthermore, the Regional Public Health Laboratories Network provided technical expertise and technical support to ASEAN member states whilst the ASEAN Risk Assessment and Risk Communication Center disseminated preventative and control measures and combating fake news. A number of ASEAN summits soon followed to agree on regional measures to fight the pandemic. These measures included an agreement to build an ASEAN stockpile of essential medical supplies and equipment and the establishment of ASEAN Recovery Fund to aid member states. The regional grouping—with a view to ensure the smooth flow of goods and strengthening supply-chain connectivity and resilience—urged member states to refrain from imposing non-tariff measures during the pandemic.

Regional efforts in combating the COVID-19 at the epidemiological level across Southeast Asia were relatively successful despite varying capacities of health systems of member states to manage the pandemic. But ASEAN members' acceptance of International Health Regulations (IHR)—an instrument of international law regarding the rights and obligations of states in handling public health emergencies—contradicted their non-conformity with international norms in areas such as the rights of migrant workers. In April 2020, the ASEAN established a COVID-19 Response Fund that sought to share best COVID-19 management practices across Southeast

Asia within the limits of ASEAN mandate of non-interference in the affairs of member states.

Conflict resolution in ASEAN is a significant contributor to the relative success of the regional grouping. The Indonesian notion of *musyawarah* (consultation) and *muafakat* (consensus) is apparent in decision-making at the regional level to prevent discord among member states. The inputs of all ASEAN member states are factored into policy-making, regardless of their population size or level of economic development.[77] Although Indonesia is the most populous ASEAN member, by surrendering its role as regional leader, differences of opinion within the regional grouping are circumvented. On the contrary, as India's South Asian neighbors perceive India as the regional hegemon, the SAARC was never conceived to settle bilateral disputes. When SAARC was established in 1985, many within Indian policy circles saw this as an attempt by smaller South Asian states to gain diplomatic leverage against India whereas Pakistan was apprehensive of an India-dominated SAARC.

The COVID-19 crisis revealed the weaknesses of a regional approach to the pandemic in South Asia. Although India proposed the SAARC COVID-19 Emergency Fund on March 13, 2020 to assist its South Asian neighbors in meeting their immediate expenses related to the pandemic, differences between India and Pakistan regarding disbursement of the fund stymied effective cooperation. Whereas India proposed the administration of the Emergency Fund as a standalone activity outside the SAARC's timetable to avoid the bureaucratic grind of the SAARC Secretariat, Pakistan intended to utilize the mechanism of the SAARC Secretariat to disburse the Emergency Fund. Differences between India and Pakistan related to the administration of the Emergency Fund were indicative of the latter's apprehension of an India-centric orientation of the regional grouping. India supported the development of a SAARC Disaster Management Center (SDMC)-managed online COVID-19 Information Exchange Platform. The online platform intended to provide timely updates about the evolving pandemic across South Asia. Since its founding in 2005, the SDMC has devised guidelines for national-level disaster management but has been struggling to implement these guidelines due to staffing issues and compelling inter-state and intra-state politics in South Asia. Additionally, unlike other regional bodies, the SDMC receives negligible external funding as South Asian countries want to protect SAARC from external interests, particularly China and the US. These factors inhibit the Center's ability to monitor member states' implementation of disaster management guidelines. Unlike ASEAN, the SAARC has not implemented the standardization of IHR guidelines at the regional level.

The second surge of COVID-19 across South Asia in April 2021 revealed why a regional approach to global health was imperative. The uncontrolled spread of the second wave implied that newer coronavirus variants would continue to emerge, display increasing transmissibility or evade vaccinations, making it difficult for states to act upon them. As SAARC member states' capacities for scaling up genomics and rolling out country-wide surveillance systems are limited, regional collaboration modeled on the lines of the Indian SARS-CoV-2 Genome Sequencing Consortia are feasible. The proposed network can connect genomic data with clinical and public health data and can provide a comprehensive picture of circulating COVID variants.

During the second wave of the pandemic in South Asia, there was a dependency on aid from the diaspora, bilateral and humanitarian agencies to secure medical supplies, although such a measure was unsustainable. Nationalistic policies and hoarding of vaccines and bulk drugs by advanced countries during the pandemic impeded equitable access and scale-up. Under such circumstances, it is imperative that SAARC nations collaborate with each other as a bloc in studying best global practices, draw up a regional plan to ensure self-sufficiency of bulk drugs and vaccines and secure surplus vaccines from advanced countries using a combination of collective needs assessment and diplomacy. As Shashika Bandara, Soumyadeep Bhoumik, Veena Sriram et al., point out in the 2021 *British Medical Journal* editorial: "Beyond the immediate benefits of addressing the pandemic, a collective regional approach, with global knowledge-exchange collaborations, will be vital for re-imagining the global health structure with equity at its centre."[78]

Notes

1 A. T. Matthias and Saroj Jayasinghe, "Worsening Economic Crisis in Sri Lanka: Impacts on Health," *The Lancet Global Health* 10, no. 7 (2022): E959, DOI: https://doi.org/10.1016/S2214-109X(22)00234-0.

2 Paul Swartzendruber and Melissa Pavlik, "Bangladesh Conflict Brief," *The Armed Conflict Location and Event Data Project*, https://acleddata.com/2018/04/12/bangladesh-conflict-brief/.

3 Zulfiqar A. Bhutta and Samiran Nundy, "On the Brink of Conflict: The People of South Asia Deserve Better," *The British Medical Journal (BMJ) Global Health* 357 (2017): j1528, DOI: http://dx.doi.org/10.1136/bmj.j1528.

4 Ibid.

5 Aminah Mohammad Arif, "Introduction: Imaginations and Constructions of South Asia: An Enchanting Abstraction?," *South Asia Multidisciplinary Academic Journal* 10 (2014): 1–27. A similar point is also made by Sunil Khilnani. See Sunil Khilnani, *The Idea of India* (London: Penguin Books, 2012).

6 For details refer David Gilman, "The Historiography of India's Partition: Between Civilization and Modernity," *The Journal of Asian Studies* 74, no. 1 (2015): 23–41. For a nuanced understanding of how specific experiences of colonial rule in Burma might alter our historical understandings of British imperialism in South Asia refer Jonathan Saha, "Is it in India? Colonial Burma as a 'Problem' in South Asian History," *South Asian History and Culture* 7, no. 1 (2016): 23–29. Jonathan Saha contends that despite being governed as an integral part of British India between 1885 and 1937, Burma (Myanmar since 1989) is considered as a distinct entity beyond South Asia. This is a heuristic separation indulged by both scholars of colonial India and colonial Burma and is in part a legacy of the territorial assumptions of Area Studies.

7 Arif, "Introduction: Imaginations and Constructions of South Asia."

8 Partha S. Ghosh, "An Enigma that is South Asia: India Versus the Region," *Asia-Pacific Review* 20, no. 1 (2013): 100–20.

9 For example, the Bangladesh, Bhutan, India, Nepal (BBIN) is a subregional architecture of countries in Eastern South Asia to enhance cooperation in sectors such as water resources management, power, connectivity, and infrastructure. For details see Ashish Shukla, "Sub-Regional Cooperation Under BBIN Framework: An Analysis," *Indian Council of World Affairs Issue Brief*, January 4, 2019, https://www.icwa.in/show_content.php?lang=1&level=3&ls_id=4817&lid=2833.

10 Ashis Nandy, "The Idea of South Asia: A Personal Note on Post-Bandung Blues," *Inter-Asian Cultural Studies* 6, no. 4 (2005): 541–45.

11 Benedict Anderson, *The Spectre of Comparisons: Nationalism, Southeast Asia and the World* (New York: Verso, 1998), 3. See also Christopher Bayly and Tim Harper, *Forgotten Armies: Freedom and Revolution in Southeast Asia* (London: Penguin Books, 2007).

12 Anderson, *Spectre of Comparisons*, 3.

13 See for example, Donald Emmerson, "'Southeast Asia': What's in a Name?", *Journal of Southeast Asian Studies* 15, no. 1 (1984): 1–18.

14 Anderson, *The Spectre of Comparisons*, 4.

15 Ibid., 5.

16 Emmerson, "Southeast Asia," 9.

17 Ibid.

18 See Robert Cribb, "Burma's Entry into the ASEAN: Background and Implications," *Asian Perspective* 22, no. 3 (1998): 49–62.

19 Zahid Shahab Ahmed and Musharaf Zahoor, "Afghanistan in SAARC: A Critical Assessment of Organisational Expansion," *South Asian Survey* 22, no. 2 (2018): 171–88.

20 The World Bank, "World Bank Data," The World Bank, https://data.worldbank.org/indicator/SP.POP.TOTL.

21 The World Bank, "Life Expectancy at Birth, Total (Years): East Asia and Pacific," World Bank Data, https://data.worldbank.org/indicator/SP.DYN.LE00.IN?locations=Z4.

22 Virasakdi Chongsuvivatwong, Kai Hong Phua, Mui Teng Yap et al., "Health and Health-care Systems in Southeast Asia: Diversity and Transitions," *The Lancet* 377 (2011): 429–37.

23 Ibid.

24 Richard J. Coker, Benjamin M Hunter, James W. Rudge et al., "Emerging Infectious Diseases in Southeast Asia: Regional Challenges to Control," *The Lancet* 377 (2011): 599–609.

25 Coker, Hunter, Rudge et al., "Emerging Infectious Diseases," 600.

26 Ibid., 601.

27 Ibid., 605.

28 Ibid.

29 Celia Lowe, "Viral Sovereignty: Security and Mistrust as Measures of Future Health in the Indonesian H5N1 Influenza Outbreak," *Medical Anthropology Theory* 6, no. 3 (2019): 109–32.

30 Lowe, "Viral Sovereignty," 117.

31 Ibid., 118.

32 Ibid.

33 Coker, Hunter, Rudge et al., "Emerging Infectious Diseases," 606. For a nuanced understanding of the disagreements related to viral sample sharing see also Sophal Ear, *Viral Sovereignty and the Political Economy of Pandemics: What Explains How Countries Handle Outbreaks?* (Abingdon, Oxon: Routledge, 2022), 11.

34 Bounlay Phommasack, Chuleeporn Jiraphongsa, Moe Ko Oo et al., "Mekong Basin Disease Surveillance (MBDS): A Trust-Based Network," *Emerging Health Threats Journal* 6 (2013), DOI: 10.3402/ehtj. v6i0.19944.

35 Coker, Hunter, Rudge et al., "Emerging Infectious Diseases," 605.

36 An authoritative account of the first decade of the WHO and the impact of the Cold War on the nascent organization is provided by Marcos Cueto, Theodore Brown and Elizabeth Fee. See Marcos Cueto, Theodore Brown and Elizabeth Fee, *The WHO: A History* (Cambridge: Cambridge University Press, 2019); For a biographical account of Brock Chisholm, the first Director General of the WHO (1948–53), the budgetary challenges of the WHO and his diplomatic tightrope between the US and the USSR, refer John Farley, *Brock Chisholm, the WHO and the Cold War* (Vancouver: UBC Press, 2008); For a rounded assessment of the collaboration between the US and the Soviet Union in the global eradication of smallpox refer Erez Manela, "A Pox on Your Narrative: Writing Disease Control into Cold War History," *Diplomatic History* 34, no. 10 (2010): 300–303.

37 Cueto, Brown and Fee, *The WHO*, 97; See also Randall Packard, *A History of Global Health: Interventions into the Lives of Other Peoples* (Baltimore: Johns Hopkins University Press, 2016).

38 See for example, Packard, *A History of Global Health*, 110. Packard's account of global malaria eradication alludes to but does not reflect the ways in which malaria eradication was appropriated and transformed by local political leadership. Neither does the account reflect the unevenness in the spread of modernization to developing countries. For detailed country studies of malaria eradication see for example, Kalinga Tudor Silva, *Decolonisation, Development and Disease: A Social History of Malaria in Sri Lanka* (Hyderabad: Orient BlackSwan, 2014), 184; For the Indonesian context of the global malaria eradication program see Vivek Neelakantan, "The Campaign against the Big Four Endemic Diseases and Indonesia's Engagement with the WHO during the Cold War 1950s," in *Public Health and National Reconstruction in Post-War Asia: International Influences, Local Transformations*, Liping Bu and Ka-che Yip edited (Abingdon, Oxon: Routledge, 2014), 154–74. The beginnings of malaria eradication in Indonesia between 1959 and 1965 looked good. On the contrary, the campaign suffered from financial and organizational bottlenecks attributed to Indonesia's decentralized political set-up and deteriorating US-American relations following President Soekarno's proclamation of Guided Democracy in 1957. Furthermore, the resistance of anopheline species to insecticide DDT was detected in central Java.
For a nuanced understanding of malaria eradication in India (1958–69), see Thomas Zimmer, "In the Name of World Health and Development: The World Health Organization and Malaria Eradication in India: 1949–70," in *International Organizations and Development, 1945–1990*, Marc Frey, Sönke Kunkel and Corinna Unger edited (Basingstoke: Palgrave MacMillan, 2014), 126–49.

39 See for example, Thomas Robertson, "DDT and the Cold War Jungle: American Environmental and Social Engineering in the Rapti Valley of Nepal," The *Journal of American History* (March 2018): 904–30. Malaria eradication in Nepal during the 1950s was embodied in the Rapti Valley Development Project (RVDP) that sought to use malaria eradication as the means to open new areas of the Rapti valley for agriculture. Unlike the failure of the global malaria eradication campaigns elsewhere by the 1960s, the RVDP wiped out the disease, largely attributed to the effectiveness of DDT. Yet, the project was unable to deliver on its stated mission related to economic and social leveling.

40 Elizabeth Fee, Theodore Brown and Marcos Cueto, "At the Roots of The World Health Organization's Challenges: Politics and Regionalization," *American Journal of Public Health* 106, no. 11 (2016): 1912–17; See also Manela, "A Pox on Your Narrative."

41 See also Bob Reinhardt, *The End of a Global Pox: America and the Eradication of Smallpox in the Cold War Era* (Ann Arbor: University of Michigan Press, 2015), 40.

42 Manela, "A Pox on Your Narrative," 301–2.

43 For the Chinese context see Liping Bu, "The Patriotic Movement and China's Socialist Reconstruction: Fighting Disease and Transforming Society, 1950–80," in *Public Health and National Reconstruction in Post-War Asia: International Influences, Local Transformations*, Liping Bu and Ka-che Yip edited (Abingdon, Oxon: Routledge, 2014), 34–51. Bu argues that the developmental experiences of post-War China differed significantly from postcolonial South and Southeast Asia. Unlike the WHO, the Chinese leaders viewed strengthening of the health of the entire population as critical to socialist reconstruction of the country and in turn, promoted the Patriotic Health Movement through mass mobilization of the population in preventive health work.

44 Dora Vargha, "Vaccination and the Communist State: Polio in Eastern Europe," in *The Politics of Vaccination: A Global History*, Christine Holmberg, Stuart Blume and Paul Greenough edited (Manchester: Manchester University Press, 2017), 77–98.

45 Cueto, Brown and Fee, *The World Health Organization.*

46 Philip Havik and José Pedro Monteiro, "Portugal, the World Health Organisation and the Regional Office for Africa: From Founding Member to Outcast (1948–1966)," *Journal of Imperial and Commonwealth History* (2021), DOI: 10.1080/03086534.2021.1892374.

47 Monica Saavedra, "Politics and Health at the WHO Regional Office for South East Asia: The Case of Portuguese India, 1949–61," *Medical History* 61, no. 3 (2017): 380–400.

48 Jessica Pearson-Patel, "French Colonialism and the Battle Against the WHO Regional Office for Africa," *Hygiea Internationalis* 13, no. 1 (2016): 65–80.

49 See for example, Saavedra, "Politics and Health," 382; For a broad overview of how national interests shaped the beginnings of the SEARO see Zimmer, "In the Name of World Health and Development," 132. Zimmer contends that there was broad consensus in the Indian Ministries of Health and External Affairs respectively that the country play a significant role in the WHO. First, as the Ministry of Health hoped to strengthen its own position within the state apparatus, it was hoped that the establishment of the SEARO in New Delhi would lead to more resources diverted to health than other issues. Second, it was WHO's perceived "non-political" approach that made it attractive to India. Prime Minister Nehru himself repeatedly expressed the conviction that the strictly "technical nature" of international health cooperation would create trust between nations and prevent the organization from being dominated by major political powers. Third, in 1948 as the WHO embarked on the establishment of the SEARO, Indians saw a real opportunity to exert influence on the organization as it was institutionalized.

50 Sanjoy Bhattacharya, "The World Health Organization and Global Smallpox Eradication," *Journal of Epidemiology and Community Health* 62, no. 10 (2008): 909–12.

51 S. S. Amrith, *Decolonizing International Health: India and Southeast Asia* (Basingstoke: Palgrave MacMillan, 2006), 102.

52 See for example, C. J. Lee, "Final Communiqué of the Asian-African Conference: Held at Bandung, 18–24 April 1955," *Interventions: International Journal of Postcolonial Studies* 11, no. 1 (2009): 94–102.

53 Su Lin Lewis and Carolien Stolte, "Other Bandungs: Afro-Asian Internationalisms in the Early Cold War," *Journal of World History* 30, nos. 1 and 2 (2019): 1–19; Naoko Shimuzu, "Diplomacy as Theatre: Staging the Bandung Conference of 1955," *Modern Asian Studies* 48, no. 1 (2013): 225–52.

54 Heloise Weber and Poppy Wirianto, "The Bandung Spirit and Solidarist Internationalism," *Australian Journal of International Affairs* 70, no. 4 (2016): 391–407.

55 Ibid; See also Mark Berger, "After the Third World?: History, Destiny and the Fate of Third Worldism," *Third World Quarterly* 25, no. 1 (2004): 9–39. To understand India's quest for pharmaceutical self-sufficiency and the choice for the Indian government (1953–58) between Soviet technical support or Western transnationals in building domestic capacity, refer Nasir Tyabji, "Negotiating Non-Alignment: Dilemmas Attendant on Initiating Pharmaceutical Production in India," *Technology and Culture* 53, no. 1 (2012): 37–60.

56 Lee, "Final Communiqué of the Asian-African Conference," 95; See also Neelakantan, "The Campaign Against the 'Big Four' Endemic Diseases," 158–59. The Eighth SEARO Session (1955) at Bandung, coincided with Indonesia's hosting of the Asian-African Conference. At the session, Indonesians expressed optimism that rural development through public health could serve as a medium to diffuse international tensions. At the Thirteenth SEAROs session, hosted by Indonesia at Bogor Palace, President Soekarno alluded to the "Bandung Spirit" when he stated that Indonesia was cooperating with other nations in the spirit of internationalism in eradicating disease and welcomed foreign aid, the country was capable of meeting its targets in eradicating malaria and TB with people's cooperation.

57 Jeremy Youde, "China's Health Diplomacy in Africa," *China: An International Journal* 8, no. 1 (March 2010): 151–63; See also Zhou Xun, *The People's Health: Health Intervention and Delivery in Mao's China*, 1949–83 (Montreal: McGill-Queen's University Press, 2020).

58 Xun, *The People's Health*.

59 Litsios Socrates, "The Long and Difficult Road to Alma- Ata: A Personal Reflection," *International Journal of Health Services* 32, no. 4 (2002): 709–32.

60 See for example, Gunawan Nugroho, "A Community Approach to Raising Health Standards in Central Java," in *Health by the People*, Kenneth Newell edited (Geneva: WHO, 1975).

61 For details see Socrates Litsios, "The Christian Medical Commission and the Development of the World Health Organization's Primary Healthcare Approach," *American Journal of Public Health* 94, no. 11 (2004): 1884–93.

62 For a nuanced Soviet side of the Alma Ata story on PHC, refer Anne-Emanuelle Birn and Nikolai Krementsov, "'Socialising Primary Care? The Soviet Union, WHO and the 1978 AlmaAta Conference," *BMJ Global Health* (2018): e000992, DOI: 10.1136/ bmjgh-2018-000992; See also Xun, *The People's Health*, 288.

63 Xun, *The People's Health*, 288.

64 Ibid., 289; See also Litsios, "The Long and Difficult Road to Alma- Ata."

65 Birn and Krementsov, "'Socialising Primary Care?."

66 Ibid.

67 Cueto, Brown and Fee, *The World Health Organization*, 181.

68 Ibid., 183.

69 For a comprehensive discussion refer Ben Wisner, "GOBI versus PHC: Some Dangers of Selective Primary Healthcare," *Social Science and Medicine* 23, no. 9 (1988): 963–69.

70 Ibid.

71 Cueto, Brown and Fee, *The World Health Organization*, 184.

72 Anne-Emanuelle Birn, "The Stages of International (Global) Health: Histories of Success or Success of History?", *Global Public Health* 4, no. 1 (2009): 50–68.

73 Nitsan Chorev, *The World Health Organization Between North and South* (Ithaca: Cornell University Press, 2012); For details see for example, The World Bank, *The World Development Report 1993: Investing in Health* (Oxford: Oxford University Press, 1993).

74 Anne-Emanuelle Birn, "The Stages of International (Global) Health," 61; Chorev, *The World Health Organization Between North and South*, 9.

75 Renissa Mawani, "Screening Out Diseased Bodies: Immigration, Mandatory HIV Testing and the Making of Healthy Canada," in *Medicine at the Border: Disease, Globalization and Security, 1850-Present*, Alison Bashford edited (Basingstoke: Palgrave MacMillan, 2014), 136–58; Carolyn Strange, "Postcard from Plaguetown: SARS and the Exoticization of Toronto," in *Medicine at the Border: Disease, Globalization and Security, 1850-Present*, Alison Bashford edited (Basingstoke: Palgrave MacMillan, 2014), 219–39; Tseng Yen-fen and Wu Chia-Ling, "Governing Germs from Outside and Within Borders: Controlling the 2003 SARS Risk in Taiwan," in *Health and Hygiene in Chinese East Asia: Policies and Publics in the Long Twentieth Century*, Angela Ki Che Leung and Charlotte Furth edited (Durham, NC: Duke University Press, 2010), 254–72.
    For a rare exception refer Vinh-Kim Nguyen, *The Republic of Therapy: Triage and Sovereignty in West Africa's Time of AIDS* (Durham, NC: Duke University Press, 2010). To understand the national impact of HIV/AIDS epidemic related to the access to generic drugs see Yu-Ling Huang, "HIV/AIDS Epidemic and the Politics of Access to Medicines in Thailand: A Study of the Health Impact of Globalization," in *Global Movements, Local Concerns: Medicine and Health in Southeast Asia*, Laurence Monnais and Harold Cook edited (Singapore: NUS Press, 2012), 171–206.

76 See for example, Packard, *A History of Global Health*.

77 Rajshree Jetly, "Conflict Management Strategies in ASEAN: Perspectives for SAARC," *The Pacific Review* 16, no. 1 (2003): 53–76.

78 Shashika Bandara, Soumyadeep Bhoumik, Veena Sriram et al., "Stronger Together: A New Pandemic Agenda for South Asia," *BMJ Global Health* 6 (2021): e006776, DOI: 10.1136/ bmjgh-2021-006776.

1 "The Monsoon Asia of Geographers"

The Cold War Beginnings of the WHO Regional Office for Southeast Asia (SEARO), 1948–60

Vivek Neelakantan

Introduction

In 1947, the Interim Commission of the World Health Organization (WHO) divided the world into a series of health areas, taking into consideration the prevalence of endemic and epidemic diseases and sanitary problems. Members of the Interim Commission imagined Southeast Asia as a geopolitical construct:

> The Central and Southeastern parts of Asia, together with Indonesia, i.e., the Monsoon Asia of Geographers should be considered as one epidemiological area. It would include the endemic foci of cholera and tuberculosis and territories most readily affected by that disease; also foci of plague endemic and epidemic. It is free from yellow fever but is severely affected by malaria, by fleaborne and mite borne rickettsiosis and by the ubiquitous smallpox. Most of the area suffers from the food deficiencies of the rice eaters, from a high tuberculosis morbidity and mortality in its cities and the prevalence of that disease in rural districts.[1]

The International Health Conference convened by the United Nations (UN) in New York, during the summer of 1946, drafted the Constitution of the WHO. It set up an Interim Commission of persons designated by 18 states to continue public health activities that the soon-to-be established WHO would inherit from earlier health organizations such as the League of Nations Health Organization (1920–45) and the Office International d' Hygiène Publique (International Office of Public Hygiene, 1907–46).[2]

Unprecedented delays in the ratifications of the WHO Constitution by countries obligated the Interim Commission to operate for 2 years. The WHO came into existence at a time when the activities of the United Nations Relief and Rehabilitation Administration (UNRRA)—established in 1943 to provide economic assistance to war-ravaged Europe—were terminated. The UN asked the Interim Commission to take over the health aspects of

DOI: 10.4324/9781003332060-2

the UNRRA program, and as a result, US$4.5 million of the UNRRA funds were appropriated by the Interim Commission.[3] At the First World Health Assembly (WHA, 1948), the Interim Commission recommended that priority be given to four projects: malaria, venereal diseases, TB, and maternal and child health (MCH). A project approach dominated the WHO's early relations with member states. By 1949, the nascent organization had also come to terms with escalating Cold War tensions between the US and the USSR. The agency moved closer to US foreign policy and became captive to US geopolitical interests in the world. It pursued a pragmatic course of limited objectives, accepted compromises over decolonization, and settled upon an institutionalized structure of regionalization.[4]

Chapter 11 of the WHO Constitution permits the WHA to define geographical areas in which it is desirable to establish regional organizations as an integral part of the WHO. The definition of a region has concerned geographers, anthropologists, ecologists, political scientists, and sociologists. Basic to the concept of a region is some kind of unity: geographic or cultural. For the regional health organization under the jurisdiction of the WHO, economic or political geography determines the need for unified action that transcends political boundaries. Rivers crossing through political boundaries give rise to transnational concerns. For example, the Commission for Control of Venereal Diseases among Boatmen on the Rhine was formed to cover the mobile population on the river.[5]

Decentralization logically follows regionalization. Decentralization is an organizational arrangement that may be assessed in terms of administrative efficiency. In a geographically dispersed setting such as the WHO, the formulation of workplans may be more effective through field or district offices. Between 1948 and 1951, there was considerable skepticism within the WHO headquarters about the feasibility of establishing regional offices. Among those opposed to the establishment of the WHO regional offices were the Economic and Social Council (ECOSOC) of the UN. As the Director General reminded the ECOSOC, "regionalization" would become efficient only when the scale of WHO's annual activity reached US $7,500,000 to $8,000,000.[6] The common misgivings held by WHO member states at the time against regionalization were that the regional offices impeded communication between WHO Expert Committees at Geneva—in touch with the most sophisticated health practices—and the lack of acquaintance with medical technologies in several member states. In such cases, the WHO regional offices were forced to tailor recommendations from WHO Expert Committees to suit local conditions. There was a certain resentment that WHO headquarters would become "rubber stamps" for half-baked proposals of regional offices.[7] There were questions raised with respect to placing the regional office in the dominant country of the region.[8]

Since 1995, the history of post-World War II international health has received scholarly attention. In his monograph *World Health and World Politics: The World Health Organization and the UN System*, Javed Siddiqi notes an inherent contradiction in the functioning of the WHO. Although the organization attempted to nurture a universal outlook and approach as evidenced in the introduction of the Global Malaria Eradication program (1955), the WHO was a decentralized organization. The significance of a decentralized regional structure could be understood in terms of status-quo of pre-existing international health organizations.[9] The existence of the Pan American Sanitary Bureau (PASB) meant that some regional arrangements would have to be arrived at if the US was to participate in, and contribute to, the new WHO.[10] The practical challenge faced by the WHO founders was how to bring about the integration of pre-existing regional organizations into the WHO and establish them as regional offices.[11]

Historians have characterized the WHO mass campaigns against disease during the 1950s as leading ex-colonial nations of Asia and Africa on a trajectory of modernity defined by the Western nations.[12] The political elites of Asia and Africa were fully reconciled to the modernization mission of the WHO. Within the WHA, Western nations were adamant in restricting their aid to technical assistance whereas newly independent countries led by India contended at the Second WHA (1949) that aid must be unilateral and unconditional.[13] In a similar vein, the Ceylonese delegate to the Fourth WHA (1951) complained that Southeast Asia was not receiving as much aid as was requested and urged ex-colonial powers to raise people's living standards in the region.[14]

Although Sung Lee and Randall Packard have talked about the use of military metaphors in the WHO's campaign against malaria, neither have investigated the unevenness in the spread of modernization to newly decolonized nations of Asia and Africa. Whereas India and Indonesia sought to achieve a delicate equilibrium between increased technical assistance in health and increased openness to international aid, the Philippines sought to align its health policy with prescriptions of international aid agencies.[15]

The regional histories of the WHO have received scant historical attention.[16] In his influential monograph, *Decolonizing International Health: India and Southeast Asia, 1930–65*, Sunil Amrith argues that the WHO was enthusiastically embraced by postcolonial governments because the organization provided a forum in which the ideas of progressive policy could be detached from their specific colonial context. By disseminating universal norms, the WHO could govern what it meant to speak of health policy to such an extent that public health meant something similar across states with very different political cultures.[17]

According to Amrith's line of argument, India played a leading role in shaping the post-World War II consensus on health in Southeast Asia and formed the nodal point in the network of expertise and policies—which touched some parts of Southeast Asia more than others—for a number of reasons. First, India presented an internationally important disease environment due to its size and diversity. Second, poverty-stricken India seemed to encapsulate a range of conditions, in what would come to be the underdeveloped world. Third, the openness of India to international assistance made the country an ideal testing ground for new approaches in tuberculosis and malaria control.[18] India or Indians played a greater role in shaping approaches to Asia's health problems than did the Indonesians or the Burmese who were absorbed by fundamental problems of constructing state authority amidst much violence. The relative dominance of India over the field of public health in the region owed to the fact that many more upper-caste Indians had been trained in biomedicine than their counterparts in the Dutch East Indies or in British Burma.[19] The biopolitics of international health reconciled, to an extent, "Indian aspirations" for regional leadership with a more general postcolonial fear of American dominance.[20] Although Amrith's monograph ascribes the centrality of India in shaping the WHO approach to health in Southeast Asia, the larger Cold War context and the role of the SEARO in liaising between Southeast Asian states, international aid agencies, and US technical assistance remain unexplored.

In this chapter, I argue that although India's role was pivotal to the establishment of the SEARO, programs implemented by the regional organization were shaped by Cold War concerns and nation-building in Southeast Asia. While drawing up regional health programs, the SEARO had to balance between ensuring compliance of member states with prescriptions of international aid agencies and lobbying at the WHO headquarters for increased budgetary allocation to Southeast Asia.

Cold War and the Politics of Regionalization

Although the process of founding the WHO was started by the San Francisco Conference (May 1945)—officially known by the appellation of the United Nations Conference on International Organizations—the US and the UK decided to leave out the field of health from the conference agenda. The establishment of the WHO was due to the initiative of Szeming Sze from China, Geraldo de Paula Souza from Brazil, and Karl Evang from Norway.[21] The Technical Preparatory Committee—convened in Paris, March 1946 consisting of 16 experts nominated by the Economic and Social Committee of the UN—played a dominant role in drafting the preamble of the WHO Constitution.[22] The proposals for regional health arrangements generated considerable discussion not only amidst the Technical Committee Members but also within the Interim Commission and the First WHA. Between 1948 and 1956, the newly established WHO was faced with twin challenges: (a) withdrawal of the USSR and its allies from the organization, due to differences with the US over socialized medicine; and (b) organizing regional offices in Southeast Asia and Western Pacific where the agency had to come to terms with the dissolution of European colonial empires and the birth of new nation states.

A direct repercussion of the Cold War was the Soviet withdrawal from the WHO in 1949. At the First WHA (1948), the USSR leveled criticisms against the budget and program of the Interim Commission. The Interim Commission had hurriedly created more than 15 committees. In 1947, the Commission spent $172,000 on conferences and technical committees; and expenditure on personnel amounted to $800,000 (1947) and $900,000 (1948).[23] Although Poland, the Byelorussia Soviet Socialist Republic, and the Ukraine Soviet Socialist Republic suffered disproportionately due to the German occupation during World War II, they received only $303,000 of the total WHO Interim Commission budget of US $1.2 million for 1947.[24]

N.A. Vinogradov, the Soviet Deputy Health Minister and delegate to the First WHA, contended that epidemics such as cholera were due to poverty and colonial exploitation and the lack of organization of health services in colonial and occupied territories. The Soviets alleged that the US did not recognize the inseparable links between social, economic, and health problems. During the First WHA, they denounced poor working conditions under capitalism and advocated the establishment of national health services.[25] Despite the tense political environment within the WHA, Chisholm and Andrija Štampar from Yugoslavia—who established the School of Public Health in Zagreb (1927) and were among of the founding fathers of the WHO—were hopeful that social medicine would still count among WHO's priorities.[26] Štampar contended that the WHO prioritizes the following four issues: (a) social and economic security; (b) education; (c) nutrition; and, (d) housing.[27] As Amrith noted, a social medicine perspective, if taken seriously, would involve redressing questions related to poverty, inequitable land holdings, and poor housing.[28] To avoid these politically sensitive issues that would incur opposition from the US, the WHO embarked on a narrow program of technical assistance. Technical assistance was based on the assumption that development was a matter of transferring knowledge of science and technology that would enable planners to circumvent the socio-economic realities that led to underdevelopment.[29]

The withdrawal of the USSR and its Eastern European allies by 1949 had an impact on the WHO's finances. The absent countries did not pay their assessed contributions for 1949. As a result, the WHO had to defer the settlement of an outstanding loan from the US and keep to the same budget level approved by the First WHA.[30] Chisholm pointed out that the Constitution of the WHO did not contain a provision for withdrawal of member states. He therefore claimed that the USSR and its allies were "inactive" rather than "withdrawn" members and announced that he would wait for their return to the organization.[31] The WHO attempted to use the good offices of the Indian Minister of Health, Raj Kumari Amrit Kaur—President of the First WHA—to assuage the USSR that the US was not running the WHO.[32]

Between 1948 and 1956, the WHO was captive to US national interests. In his inaugural address on January 20, 1949, President Harry Truman outlined the Point Four Program to contain the spread of Communist ideology. The agenda of the Point Four Program included unfaltering support of the UN and related agencies; strengthening world economic recovery; strengthening freedom-loving countries against the dangers of aggression; and provision of technical assistance for economically underdeveloped areas.[33] Through participation in the WHO activities, it was hoped that the US could help create conditions congenial to economic stability and sustenance of democratic institutions that included improving health and improving peoples' living standards, particularly in the underdeveloped countries that were the prime targets of Communist ideology.[34] At the time, US contributed to 40 percent of the WHO's expanded technical assistance program and about 95 percent of funding for the organization's malaria eradication program.[35]

With the death of Soviet leader Joseph Stalin (a communist hardliner) in 1953, an incipient de-Stalinization program was launched under the leadership of Nikita Khrushchev who emphasized peaceful co-existence with the US both within and outside the UN.[36] In 1955, the Soviets expressed their desire to join the WHO.[37] The WHO welcomed the re-entry of the USSR and its allies and requested it to repay only a small percentage of its assessed contributions.[38]

Apart from Cold War rivalries, the newly established WHO had to come to terms with regionalization. The form of decentralization that the WHO took was the establishment of regional organizations rather than administrative decentralization. This form of decentralization was dictated by the circumstances of the time, particularly by the insistence of Latin American states on preserving the autonomy of the PASB. The Constitution of the WHO states that the WHA shall from time to time define geographical areas in which it is desirable to establish regional organizations. The WHA may—with the consent of a majority of members situated within each area so defined—establish a regional organization to meet the special needs of such areas.[39] The WHO Constitution does not mention any criteria that can be applied for delineating geographical areas.

Within the Interim Commission, there was considerable debate about the immediate need to define geographical areas and the desirability of establishing regional organizations until the central organization was firmly established. The USSR recommended the "absorption" of the PASO and other pre-existing regional organizations into the WHO whereas no such drastic solution was acceptable to the US.[40] The US delegation to the Interim Commission, led by Thomas Parran, submitted a draft resolution to the effect that pre-existing regional health agencies be brought into special relationship with the WHO through special arrangements and that such agencies be transformed into regional offices.

The Indian delegates impressed on the Interim Commission the need for early regionalization.

Chapter 11, Article 44 of the WHO Constitution makes it incumbent for the WHA to have a regional set up. After a somewhat animated discussion at the First WHA, three Working Parties were appointed to make recommendations with respect to three regions: Southeast Asia, Far East, and the Middle East.[41] Each working party consisted of members from interested countries of that region. Pakistan was originally nominated to the Working Party for the Southeast Asian region but was transferred to the Working Party for the Middle East with the support of the Egyptian delegate because of the former's interest to join the Middle East. Pakistan therefore did not take part in the deliberations of the Southeast Asian Working Party.[42]

The First WHA defined six geographical areas. Three of them—Southeast Asia, Eastern Mediterranean, and West Pacific—were defined by enumeration of member states. Two areas—Europe and the Americas—were delineated by reference to a continental mass. Africa was defined by referring to its natural and political boundaries. Between 1948 and 1953, there was a lack of consensus within the WHA on assignment of member states to regional organizations.[43] The WHO Executive Board in order to implement the recommendations of the First WHA (1948) approved the establishment of the SEARO on January 1, 1949. The Board conditionally approved the selection of Delhi as the site of the Regional Office for Southeast Asia, subject to the consultation of the WHO Director General with the UN.[44]

Newly independent India and the Philippines influenced the WHA's thinking on regionalization. Amrit Kaur—India's chief delegate to the Second WHA—argued that for its institutional growth, the WHO should not rely exclusively on committees, questionnaires, and paperwork. The salvation of backward countries and their sound development was the key to world health. In emphasizing India's rural character and widespread poverty, she exhorted the WHO to concentrate its activities on environmental sanitation. She also noted that without regional offices, the implementation of WHO's field programs would be jeopardized.[45] In a similar vein, A. Villarama, the Health Secretary of the Philippines stated that the WHO programs should be tailored to local conditions. He sketched a dark picture of disease by stating to the effect that one Filipino died of TB every 15 minutes to increase WHO funding for the Philippines for the control of communicable diseases.[46]

The Philippines had aspired to establish the headquarters for the would-be WHO Regional Office for the Western Pacific (WPRO) at Manila. In justifying his country's location for the WHO regional office, Villarama argued:

> I believe that the Philippine position is unique: it cannot be considered properly as one with India, because of its great distance from that vast country; it is, geographically and commercially, the hub of the wheel in the Far East, Australia and New Zealand being far down south in the Western Pacific Area, and thus being not quite disposed to join hands with us in the consideration of the establishment of a regional organization in that area, with headquarters in the Philippines.[47]

The beginnings of the WPRO were delayed because Australia and New Zealand did not want to commit themselves to establishing the regional organization. There was little commonality between the northern and southern portions of what had been designated as the WPRO. The WHO Executive Board eventually decided in 1950 to establish an administrative office for the Western Pacific region even though the consent of a majority of the members of the Western Pacific had not been obtained.[48]

Before the end of 1951, regional organizations were established in the six geographical areas delineated by the First WHA. Article 46 of the WHO Constitution stipulates that each regional organization shall consist of a regional office and a regional committee. Article 47 states that regional committees shall be composed of representatives of member states and Associate Members. The Second WHA (1949) defined members in a region as those states which had the seat of government within the region. On the contrary, the WHA defined Associate Members as those states that did not have the seat of government within the region but either by the reason of their constitution considered a certain territory or groups of territories in the region as a part of their natural territory or were responsible for the conduct of the international relations of the territory or groups of territories. Associate Members were permitted to participate in the deliberations of the regional committee but were not allowed to vote in plenary meetings of the regional committee.[49]

The inclusion of the Netherlands as an Associate Member representing its colonial interests in Indonesia in the regional body for Southeast Asia was complicated due to the partitioning of the region into the SEARO and the would-be WPRO.[50] In 1948, the Department of Health of the Dutch East Indies (Departemen van Gezondheid) had expressed a serious reservation that the newly constituted SEARO would be of limited benefit to Indonesia as Batavia (now known as Jakarta) was geographically closer to the would-be WHO Regional Office for the Western Pacific at Manila than New Delhi.[51] But India supported the revolutionary government—then headquartered at Yogyakarta (1948)—to accede to the SEARO. At the Third WHA (1950), the US of Indonesia decided not to accede to the West Pacific Region—as was taken in the First WHA—but to the Southeast Asia area.[52]

At the First WHA, India, Ceylon (now Sri Lanka), Burma (Myanmar since 1989), Siam (Thailand), and Afghanistan consented to join the SEARO. Between 1949 and 1953, France (representing the territory of Pondicherry), Portugal (representing its possessions in Goa and Daman and Diu), and the UK (representing the Maldives) were permitted to participate in the SEARO regional deliberations as Associate Members. Vietnam, Cambodia, and Laos were provisionally assigned to the SEARO at the time of the Third WHA (1950) but when the WPRO was established in 1951, these three countries acceded to that regional office.[53] In 1969, Afghanistan—a SEARO founder member—transferred at its own request to the EMRO (WHO Regional Office for the Eastern Mediterranean) due to geographical contiguity with the Middle East and for political reasons.[54]

The criteria for assigning individual countries to WHO regional offices remained ambiguous until 1959. The USSR—upon its readmission to the

WHO in 1956—invoked Article 47 of the WHO Constitution to secure Associate Membership in the SEARO. The Soviet delegate to the Twelfth World Health Assembly (1959) contended that the five Soviet republics (Uzbek, Tadzhik, Turkmenian, Kazakh, and Kirghiz) were situated in the Asiatic portion of the country and were directly contiguous to Afghanistan. The geographical proximity of the Soviet republics to the SEARO member state of Afghanistan led the USSR to have an interest in joint solutions to health problems of Southeast Asia.[55] But the Twelfth WHA deferred the proposed Soviet Union's Associate Membership of the SEARO on the grounds that the five Soviet republics were contiguous with the USSR and were not constitutionally self-governing countries situated within Southeast Asia.[56] The USSR subsequently withdrew its proposal.

The Early Years of the SEARO: Setting up Health Agendas and Tackling Endemic Diseases, 1948–60

Between 1948 and 1951, the SEARO's priorities were congruent with those emphasized by the First WHA at Geneva. The regional organization emphasized the "Big Six" that included malaria, TB, venereal diseases, maternal and child health (MCH), nutrition, and environmental sanitation. The SEARO's technical assistance for member states was focused on developing 2-year short-term demonstration projects. Such projects entailed selection of several areas within Southeast Asia that included: (a) a combined attack on health problems affecting the community; and (b) development of a comprehensive program of educating the community on the rational application of public health methods. Early SEARO support for member states focused on the organization of mass campaigns against malaria, tuberculosis, and yaws. But by 1951 the SEARO redirected its priority to long-term technical assistance to member states and training of health personnel. By 1960, two public health approaches became apparent in the programs of the SEARO: (a) the proverbial magic bullet approach that focused on the eradication of disease; and (b) a more holistic approach that linked public health to broader social questions such as poverty. The regional office aggregated requests from member states for technical assistance. The meeting of country-specific requests and tailoring the recommendations of the WHO Expert Committees to local conditions formed the backbone of the SEARO programs.

The First SEARO Regional Committee Meeting was inaugurated by the Indian Prime Minister Jawaharlal Nehru on October 4, 1948. The Meeting was attended by delegates from India, Ceylon, Siam, Afghanistan, and Burma who unanimously approved the nomination of Lieutenant Colonel Chandra Mani (1903–78) from India as the Regional Director of the SEARO. C. Mani served as the Regional Director between 1948 and 1968. After completing medical training in the UK, he served in the Indian Medical Service (1927–36) as Deputy Assistant Director of Hygiene (1939–43), and subsequently as the Deputy Director General of Health, Government of India (1947–48).[57] Prior to his appointment as Deputy Director General of Health, C. Mani served as Director of Public Health of the state of Orissa and subsequently as the Deputy Public Health Commissioner of Delhi. C. Mani and Sze presented a joint proposal to the Technical Preparatory Committee for the regionalization of the would-be WHO.[58] C. Mani noted that the relationship between the Headquarters of the would-be WHO and the regional organizations was as follows: the former being assigned general functions with respect to quarantine and epidemiological intelligence gathering whereas the latter organization, regional functions such as rural sanitation and village water supplies.

The SEARO regional health program—that commenced operations from January 1, 1949—aggregated requests from member states. During the first year of the regional organization, India requested for help in combating malaria, TB, venereal diseases, and MCH. The SEARO's first work in the region was in the field of TB control and it assisted the governments of India and Ceylon in setting up BCG campaigns.[59] In the field of malaria control, the SEARO awarded fellowships that enabled two medical officers from Thailand and one from Ceylon to undertake a 3-month course at the National Institute of Malariology in India.[60] In 1949, the regional organization also assisted the Indian government in setting up four malaria demonstration control teams.[61] The following year, the SEARO team undertook a malarial survey in Afghanistan that led to the establishment of a malaria demonstration project in Laghman, Jalalabad province.[62] In both malaria demonstration projects, the SEARO sourced supplies of insecticide DDT from the UNICEF.

In India, the malaria demonstration projects were located in the Western Terai district of United Provinces (now Uttar Pradesh), Jeypore hill tracts of Orissa, Malnad region of Mysore, and Ernad region of Malabar. The Terai was jointly selected by the SEARO and the FAO because the rich agricultural potentiality of the area was arrested due to malaria. With a view to open the Terai for agriculture, the Indian government encouraged the resettlement of Hindu and Sikh Punjabi families in the Terai who were earlier displaced by partition (1947). Malaria control was undertaken in the Western Terai between May and July 1949.[63] With the assistance of public health nurses, attempts were made to extend maternal and child care in certain parts of the Terai.

Cora Du Bois—a cultural anthropologist, head of the US State Department's Southeast Asia Branch who was later hired by the WHO between 1950 and 1951—was critical of the SEARO's malaria demonstration project in Terai. She noted that the local population, particularly the Buxas, did not cooperate with the anti-malarial spraying squads for fear of getting dispossessed from their lands.[64] In her letter to C. Mani, Du Bois recommended that the SEARO reassess the narrowly defined demonstration projects for disease control.[65] Du Bois warned

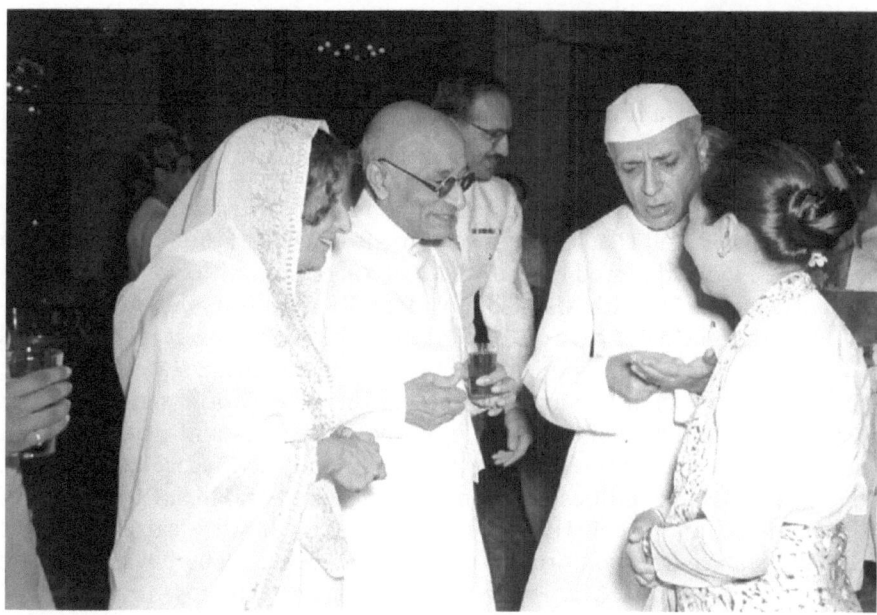

Figure 1.1 A reception held by Rajkumari Amrit Kaur, India's Minister of Health in honor of SEARO Conference delegates at Government House, New Delhi on September 27, 1949.

A reception was held by Indian Minister of Health Rajkumari Amrit Kaur at Government House, Delhi (September 27, 1949), in honor of delegates to the SEARO Conference. From left to right: Amrit Kaur, C. Rajagopalachari (India's Last Governor General), Indian Premier Jawaharlal Nehru, and Madam Aung San (Director of Women's and Children's Welfare Board, Burma).

Photo Credit: Photo 11245, Public.Resource.Org
Studio/Oct 49, A 22 p
https://www.flickr.com/photos/publicresourceorg/27081104530/in/album-72157669011055206/

that instead of trying to slip MCH goals into the malaria demonstration project, which would produce inferior results, the SEARO should concentrate on training local health personnel.[66] Although Mani did not reply to her letters, by 1951 there was acknowledgment within the SEARO that the 2-year short-term demonstration projects were unsustainable. The Regional Committee, instead, redirected its efforts toward long-term assistance to member states, that included the training of health personnel.

Malaria was endemic in most areas of Afghanistan in 1949. In 1950, the SEARO set up malaria control operations in Laghman (near Jalalabad) and in Kunduz and trained local health personnel in anti-malarial operations. Since malaria is transmitted seasonally in Afghanistan, the National Malaria Organization was deployed to control typhus during the winter in Kabul and Kandahar.[67] The SEARO short-term demonstration project had aroused the local population's interest in malaria control such that the government was unable to cope with the increased demand to expand the malaria control operations to all areas of the country.[68] By 1954, the transmission of malaria in Afghanistan was intercepted with only one round of spraying as the vectors *Anopheline superpictus* and *Anopheline culcifacies* were susceptible to DDT.[69]

US Epidemiologist Robert Briggs Watson had served as a field member of the International Health Division of the Rockefeller Foundation between 1942 and 1966 and served on the WHO's Expert Committee on Malaria. In his correspondence with Malariologist Paul Russell, Watson noted (as early as 1950) that the early part of the SEARO work in India was characterized by ill-will toward the organization.[70] For example, in the state of Mysore, the state government had anticipated that the WHO would send a malaria team that would be self-sufficient in terms of finances and personnel. But due to a lack of coordination between Delhi and the Mysore government, the lines of responsibilities between the central and provincial governments on one hand and the WHO were not demarcated. All local expenses of SEARO staff had to be borne by state governments.[71] There was a certain resentment toward C. Mani at the state level as he was close to the central government at New Delhi.[72]

Although the SEARO short-term demonstration projects were not unsuccessful, the health authorities of most countries had neither the means nor the manpower to expand the projects on a countrywide basis. In a letter to the WHO Headquarters on May 11, 1949, C. Mani pointed out that attention to sanitation would have a decisive effect in the control and eventual elimination of diseases such as ancylostomiasis, typhoid, and cholera (then prevalent in Madras and Bengal).[73] He noted that basic requirements for control of cholera such as wholesome water supply and sanitary disposal of excreta were woefully inadequate throughout the Southeast Asia region. C. Mani liaised the SEARO member states with the WHO headquarters for technical assistance in health.

Apart from the WHO Headquarters, C. Mani liaised with the US technical authorities, beginning March 1950. Representatives of the US Public Health Service called on the Regional Director to discuss the ways in which technical assistance could be provided to countries of Southeast Asia under the Point Four Program.[74] The Colombo Plan for Southeast Asia was founded in 1950 by the governments of Australia, the UK, New Zealand, and Canada at a meeting held in Colombo. Although the bulk of technical assistance under the Colombo Plan was allocated to industrial and agricultural development in South and Southeast Asia, support was also given to training medical and paramedical personnel through fellowships.[75] During the early years of the SEARO, public health programs in the region were ad hoc and donor-driven. As early as December 1951, C. Mani proposed to the WHO Headquarters and secured approval for the appointment of WHO Area Representatives for each member state. These representatives worked under the supervision of the Regional Director and provided advice to governments on health planning.[76]

On October 31, 1951, at the Second General Session of the American Public Health Association, C. Mani outlined the challenges faced by the nascent regional organization:

> The Southeast Asia Region of the World Health Organization comprises Afghanistan, Burma, Ceylon, India, Indonesia, and Thailand. It contains nearly 500 million people—more than three times the population of the United States in less than three-fourths of that area. The population is very unevenly distributed, with some areas very heavily populated, such as the Ganges valley and Java; but there are also large areas with very few people. More than 80 per cent of the people live in villages, 80 per cent are illiterate and the average income is in the neighborhood of $50. All public health planning must start with these facts.[77]

Health conditions of the region were shaped by communicable diseases such as smallpox, cholera, typhoid, and endemic diseases such as malaria and tuberculosis. C. Mani contended that chronic poverty and malnutrition had sapped people's desire for improvement. He noted that even though the WHO had the resources to launch large-scale disease eradication campaigns, SEARO member states would be unable to sustain the efforts of the WHO after overseas assistance ended.[78] The SEARO had concentrated its activities in a few well-chosen public health fields to avoid the dispersion of scarce resources.

At the Third WHA (1950), of the total WHO annual budget of US$7.3 million, US$682,000 was allocated to the SEARO by the Director General, Brock Chisholm, under Technical Assistance.[79] The UNICEF provided equipment for health programs for which the WHO had given its approval. Between 1951 and 1955, the WHO and the UNICEF supported the BCG campaign in India.[80] India's First Five-Year Plan (1951–56) gave top priority to BCG.[81] The Indian chapter of the BCG campaign was complicated due to administrative fault lines and resistance to BCG, particularly in the Madras state spearheaded by the then Chief Minister C. Rajagopalachari (1952–54).[82] The other reason for resistance to BCG was the general distrust of international organizations. BCG vaccinations were associated with birth control, particularly in the populous state of Uttar Pradesh.[83] In 1959, for example, a rumor circulated that teams of doctors were moving about the country injecting poison into the blood of people to keep the population down.[84]

The mass campaign against TB was implemented in Delhi (February 23, 1953) in commemoration of BCG Day and inaugurated by Rajkumari Amrit Kaur. The photo depicts a baby receiving the BCG vaccine.

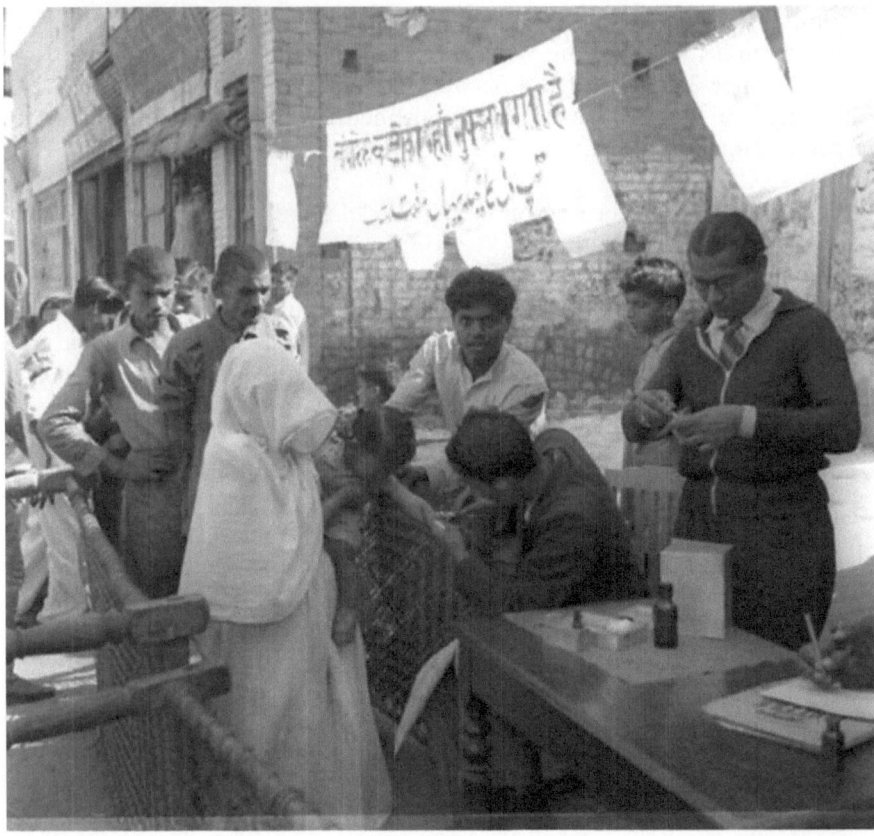

Figure 1.2 A mass campaign against TB, implemented in Delhi on February 23, 1953, in commemoration of BCG day. A small baby receiving the BCG vaccine.

Photo Credit: Internet Library Public Resource, Photo No. 32077
https://archive.org/details/propix.27506850185

In Indonesia, the SEARO operated a pilot TB Control and Demonstration Center in Bandung, West Java province (1952–57), to investigate the prevalence of TB and suggest prevention measures. In 1952—when the project was first implemented—the city of Bandung was facing an acute shortage of hospital beds. The SEARO recommended ambulatory chemoprophylaxis—*mantris* (nurses) visiting patients' homes and educating families about the contagiousness of TB, administering drugs such as streptomycin and isoniazid, isolating infected patients and their contacts, and ensuring that patients continued their medication.[85] The project was beset with administrative bottlenecks. The project was administered by the TB Section of the Indonesian Ministry of Health but was devolved to the Inspectorate of Health, West Java in 1954. But the Bandung municipal authorities were not involved due to lack of finances. The then Indonesian Minister of Health Johannes Leimena sought to integrate tuberculosis control within the framework of basic health services under the so-called Bandung Plan for Health (introduced in 1951) but the plan was somewhat overambitious due to lack of finances. Not surprisingly, the project suffered from staffing issues that impeded the detection, effective treatment, and follow-up of TB patients and their contacts.

During its first 3 years, the SEARO confined its activities to the establishment of 2-year short-term demonstration projects for the control of communicable diseases. At the same time, India disembarked on the First Five-Year Plan (1951–56). The First Five Year Plan stated that the improvement of public health was often a matter of imparting elementary knowledge regarding sanitation and hygiene.[86] In 1952, Burma launched its first welfare plan entitled *Pyidawtha* (Prosperous Royal Country). The Plan was inclusive of transfer of power to local governments, health education, economy, nationalization of arable lands, infrastructural development, self-sufficiency, democratically elected local councils, development of frontier areas, and national reconstruction.[87] Prime Minister U Nu's pledge was to bring to each Burmese a brick house, a car, and 800 kyats in salary. The use of the word *Pyidawtha* signified the coalescence between the Prime Minister's promise of national development and the preservation of Burmese traditions. The Plan also reflected U Nu's confident start to rebuild the country after ethnic strife that devastated the country following civil war (1948). The SEARO's ability in fulfilling its aspirations of assisting member states in building their health infrastructures during the 1950s was curtailed due to the reduction in the UN Technical Assistance program budget. For the financial year 1953, the SEARO regional budget, amounting to US$2 million was slashed to US$900,000.[88]

In the SEARO Annual Reports, C. Mani frequently complained about the reductions in the WHO annual budget for regional organizations. He expressed disappointment that as regional efforts for disease control intensified, international aid trailed off for communicable diseases.[89] In February 1953, the Technical Cooperation Administration (TCA) of the Eisenhower administration and the WHO Headquarters organized a Joint Staff Conference that included the Regional Directors of the EMRO, SEARO, and WPRO. At the conference, C. Mani emphasized that US assistance for Southeast Asia could be directed to malaria control and the need for SEARO to liaise with TCA before granting requests for medical assistance from countries of the region.[90] Furthermore, C. Mani urged the TCA to recruit regional staff who would, in turn, liaise with SEARO Area Representatives in formulating a regional health plan. He was disappointed as neither the SEARO nor the TCA had adequately addressed the question of environmental sanitation in Southeast Asia. Although the TCA had introduced a sanitation component in the community development projects across Southeast Asia that it was assisting, C. Mani urged the aid agency to prioritize safe drinking water. He noted that the TCA plan of building hospitals across Southeast Asia was unwise as some governments of the region had inadequate resources even for running existing hospitals.

Foreign aid was a sensitive issue in Southeast Asian politics during the 1950s. Leaders of India, Ceylon, Indonesia, and Burma had to tread a delicate tightrope between preserving their country's political sovereignty and increasing receptivity to overseas technical assistance. The Asian-African Conference—more popularly known by the appellation of Bandung Conference, hosted by Indonesia at Bandung in April 1955—discussed problems of common concern to Asia and Africa. The Conference discussed ways in which leaders of newly independent countries of both continents could achieve fuller economic, cultural, and political cooperation. Indonesia hosted the Eighth SEARO Regional Conference in September 1955 at Bandung. The Communiqué of the Asian-African Conference influenced the agenda of the SEARO in 1955.

The Communiqué of the Asian-African Conference emphasized economic cooperation of participating Asian and African countries based on mutual interest and respect for national sovereignty. Participating countries agreed to provide technical assistance to one another, to the maximum extent practicable, in the form of experts, trainees, pilot projects, exchange of technical knowhow, and establishment of national and regional training institutes for imparting technical skills in cooperation with existing regional agencies.[91] Although health was not explicitly mentioned on the agenda of the Asian-African Conference, the Communiqué expressed concerns about the looming Cold War tensions and the dangers of an atomic war.[92] The Communiqué exhorted all states to bring about a reduction of armaments, eliminate of nuclear weapons and harness nuclear energy for peaceful purposes. Global peace would help answer the needs, particularly of Asia and Africa, and particularly in social progress and better standards of life.

Inaugurating the Eighth Regional SEARO Conference, Leimena discussed common concerns broached by leaders of Asia and Africa, including raising people's living standards. Leimena's opening address articulated a holistic perspective of health that was at odds with the proverbial magic bullet approach which gained currency in international health during the mid-1950s. He contended that communicable disease was the result of an interaction of a triad: with humans as the primary concern; the agent of the disease; and, environmental, social, and biological variables. The ecology of disease needed to be taken into account by governments while engineering public health measures. He acknowledged that the top priorities for SEARO member states included environmental sanitation, health education, and adequate training of health personnel.[93] Leimena exhorted the SEARO to redress health problems of the region by taking into account people's living conditions.

Between 1948 and 1957, SEARO field programs for improving environmental health and sanitation, including the provision of safe drinking water, began initially as a part of malaria control and rural health demonstration projects. Progress in the field of environmental sanitation was slow in the region due to the inadequacy of trained personnel and shortage of overseas funding. US politics undermined global hygiene initiatives, including the SEARO programs in Southeast Asia. In 1951, President Truman established the Mutual Security Agency (MSA)—under the provisions of the Mutual Security Act—that authorized the US to provide military, technological, and economic assistance to friendly states.[94] In 1953, the Eisenhower administration replaced the MSA by the Foreign Operations Administration (FOA). These shifts hampered US overseas development assistance in significant ways and tied it to uncoordinated economic, social, political, and military objectives and programs.[95] Efforts to get American public health workers to get involved in international health were undermined by right-wing elements in America, led by J. Edgar Hoover. For instance, when Du Bois joined the WHO, Hoover ordered the FBI to conduct a thorough investigation on her.[96]

The failure of rural health in Southeast Asia did not impact the progress of the malaria control program. If anything, American Cold War imperatives greatly strengthened the resolution for malaria eradication in the region. During the early 1950s, it was widely held that malaria elimination in the region was possible due to the success of large-scale application of the insecticide DDT. The beginnings of malaria elimination looked promising, particularly in Afghanistan and Indonesia. But the mid-1950s, in Indonesia and the Akyab coast of Burma, the vector species *Anopheles sundaicus* had developed resistance to DDT.[97] By 1955, in response to vector resistance to the insecticide DDT, malaria eradication was adopted as the goal of SEARO member states.[98] In 1956, UNICEF agreed to support malaria eradication programs in Burma and Afghanistan whereas India and Indonesia disembarked on national malaria eradication programs in 1958 and 1959, respectively. The ICA (International Cooperation Administration, a US governmental agency operational between 1955 and 1961) assisted India and Indonesia with supplies of DDT.

In 1959, President Soekarno inaugurated the Indonesian chapter of the malaria eradication program in collaboration with the ICA. In his opening address, Soekarno substituted the word malaria with mal-mosquito to emphasize that malaria was not dictated by tropical climate but caused by mosquito bites that paralyzed the nation's economic potential.[99] Eradicating malaria, in Soekarno's vision, would lead to the creation of a strong and healthy Indonesian population (*rakjat sehat, negara kuat*). Indonesia aligned its nationalist rhetoric on malaria eradication with those of international agencies—that quantified economic losses sustained internationally due to the disease—to maximize US assistance. Since 1959, malaria eradication in Indonesia suffered from organizational bottlenecks associated with bureaucratic procedures that had to be followed by the malaria eradication staff at the central, provincial, and local levels, for requesting accessories and DDT supplies. As a consequence, the program made slow progress between 1959 and 1960 that led to a halving of ICA funding for the country's eradication program.[100] The ICA made a direct appeal to the then Indonesian Prime Minister Djuanda to slow down the program whereas the Indonesian Minister of Health Satrio was fighting to expand coverage. As the SEARO Regional Director, C. Mani was faced with the delicate task of ensuring compliance of the Indonesian Ministry of Health with ICA directives while granting autonomy to the National Malaria Eradication Program in line with Satrio's objective.

By 1957, the SEARO advocated a merger of MCH, communicable disease control, work for the improvement of environmental sanitation, nutrition, and health education within the broad framework of community development and rural health services. At the same time, the organization conducted a Rural Health Conference in New Delhi to discuss problems of organizing health services in rural areas. Key themes discussed at the conference included the exchange of technical information on the state of rural health services in each SEARO member state, organization and administration of rural health services, training of health personnel, and community participation in rural health.[101]

The first reason inhibiting the development of rural health services across Southeast Asia was the lack of demarcation of responsibilities between governments of member states and the SEARO with respect to management of the health demonstration projects. Second, during the 1950s, given their budgetary limitations, Southeast Asian nations focused on symbolic disease eradication campaigns rather than rural health problems.[102] The Soekarno administration, for example, focused on the "Big Four Endemic Diseases," that vitiated the overall productive capacity of the population. These diseases included malaria, TB, yaws, and leprosy. At the Thirteenth Annual Meeting of the SEARO (Bandung, 1960), C. Mani cautioned member states that although Southeast Asia had registered considerable improvements in reducing mortality attributed to communicable diseases, the main cause of morbidity in the region included malnutrition and environmental sanitation.[103] He indicated that the SEARO could assist member states in planning projects related to environmental sanitation but actual implementation of the projects would be contingent on governments' capacity to obtain adequate finances.

Despite official hype about rural health projects across SEARO member states, in reality, the decade beginning 1960 saw a perceptible decline in rural health programs. At the Thirteenth SEARO Annual Meeting, Soekarno expressed Indonesia's hesitancy in accepting foreign aid in health, and instead, advocated self-help.[104] Burma rejected foreign aid altogether with the proclamation of the "Burmese Way to Socialism," subsequent to military takeover of the country in 1962.[105] The rejection of outside help would change in the 1970s when Indonesia and Burma secured overseas developmental assistance—particularly from Japan—as both countries disembarked on a program of economic liberalization.

Conclusion: A "Southeast Asian Approach to Health" Pioneered by the SEARO?

In *Decolonizing International Health*, Amrith observes that there was a remarkable similarity in health policies adopted by polities as different as those of Indonesia, India, and Burma framed within a broad "Southeast Asian Approach to Health."[106] Across South and Southeast Asia, each state had a malaria control organization; each undertook a mass BCG vaccination against TB, and each followed the lead of the WHO, although in none of these political cultures was public health anything like a priority in government spending and public policy.[107] It is unclear as to whether the broad "Southeast Asian Approach to Health" was an outcome of the Asian-African Conference that gave rise to the Bandung Spirit that advocated a non-aligned foreign policy, solidarity with decolonized nations in a similar economic position, and economic self-sufficiency.[108] Or, did the SEARO embody a distinctive Southeast Asian approach to health?

It could be argued that during the 1950s, there were few truly regional WHO programs apart from the Fellowships Programs. Between 1948 and 1950, the SEARO offered fellowships to medical officers from Burma, Thailand, Ceylon, Portuguese India (Goa since 1961), and India to study malaria control problems at the Malaria Institute of India that would soon become a regional training center.

The first SEARO programs represented an aggregation of member states' request for technical assistance. During its early years, the SEARO was less concerned with the development of a balanced regional program than with presenting country requests for technical assistance. There was negligible effort on the part of the regional body to consider health programs in the light of other aid agencies or the country's ability to absorb international aid. During the 1950s, the Regional Committee learnt by trial and error the ways in which the WHO assistance could be meaningfully applied to suit local requirements. For example, whereas it was possible for the SEARO to award fellowships for national health staff to undertake special training within the region, it was difficult for the SEARO to influence local circumstances of member states such that fellows could apply the skills gained from regional training to work in local settings.

Since 1953, the SEARO interpreted guidelines issued by the WHO Headquarters while considering requests of individual member states for WHO assistance—although countries of the region faced difficulties in delineating their health priorities or implementing WHO guidelines. The difficulty could be partly attributed to the aspirations of postcolonial states in meeting the rising demands of the population with limited resources. At the same time, Western donors—with their own specific ideas of technical assistance—thrust aid on newly independent states of Southeast Asia without taking into account recipient nations' capacity to absorb foreign aid and continue the sponsored program once aid was discontinued. Although bilateral aid from the Western bloc to Southeast Asian nations was larger than the UN program of technical assistance, out of necessity such aid had political or economic strings attached to it. Overseas donors would not consult the WHO or other UN agencies while administering developmental assistance to Southeast Asia, leading to lopsided aid programs. In such situations, the SEARO sought to steer public health priorities of member states in the direction of what would be reasonably attainable instead of what would be desirable.

Acknowledgments

Data collection for the chapter was made possible due to a generous travel grant from the Consortium for the History of Science, Technology, and Medicine, sponsored by the Wellcome Trust (2018–19). I thank Professor Liping Bu for her encouragement and intellectual inputs that strengthened the chapter.

Notes

1 WHO Interim Commission, "Delimitation of Regional Health Areas on an Epidemiological Basis," March 31, 1947, Doc. WHO.IC/61 (Rev. 1), Subject 452, Series 1, File 5, Archives of the WHO, Geneva (henceforth WHOA).
2 For details related to the history of international health in Southeast Asia prior to 1945, refer to Lenore Manderson, "Wireless Wars in the Eastern Arena: Epidemiological Surveillance, Disease Prevention and the Work of the Eastern Bureau of the League of Nations Health Organisation, 1925–42," in *International Health: Organisations and Movements, 1925–42*, edited by Paul Weindling (Cambridge: Cambridge University Press, 1995), 109–33. See also Marcos Cueto, Theodore Brown and Elizabeth Fee, *The World Health Organization: A History* (Cambridge: Cambridge University Press, 2019). The monograph provides a comprehensive account of the continuities and changes between pre-World War II and post-World War II international health.
3 Charles S. Ascher, "Current Problems in the WHO's Program," *International Organization* 6, no. 1 (1952): 27–50.
4 See also Elizabeth Fee, Marcos Cueto and Theodore Brown, "At the Roots of World Health Organization's Challenges: Politics and Regionalization," *American Journal of Public Health* 106, no. 11 (2016): 1912–17.
5 Ascher, "Current Problems," 34.
6 Ibid., 35.
7 Ibid.
8 Ibid., 37.
9 Javed Siddiqi, *World Health and World Politics: World Health Organization and the UN System* (London: Hurst and Co., 1995), 54–55.
10 See also Marcos Cueto, *The Value of Health: A History of the Pan American Health Organization* (Washington, DC: PAHO, 2006).
11 For understanding the influence of decolonization on the establishment of WHO regional offices in the context of Africa, see Jessica Pearson-Patel,

"French Colonialism and the Battle against the WHO Regional Office for Africa," *Hygiea Internationalis* 13, no. 1 (2016): 65–80. The future AFRO faced competition from Commission for Technical Cooperation in Africa to the South of the Sahara (CTCA) by British and French governments to discuss possible technical cooperation in health between their colonial empires. The CTCA was focused more on sharing technical expertise between African colonies rather than global perspectives on health and bilateral cooperation within the framework of technical assistance that the WHO advocated.

12 Sung Lee, "WHO and the Developing World: Contest for Ideology," in *Western Medicine as Contested Knowledge*, edited by Andrew Cunningham and Bridie Andrews (Manchester: Manchester University Press, 1997), 24–45. For a similar line of argument, refer Randall Packard, *A History of Global Health: Interventions into the Lives of Other Peoples* (Baltimore, MD: Johns Hopkins University Press, 2016).

13 Lee, "WHO and the Developing World," 26.

14 Ibid.

15 For a nuanced understanding of the unevenness in the spread of modernization to newly-decolonized nations see Vivek Neelakantan, *Science, Public Health and Nation-Building in Soekarno-Era Indonesia* (Newcastle-upon-Tyne: Cambridge Scholars, 2017); Vivek Neelakantan, "'No Nation Can Go Forward When it is Crippled by Disease:' Philippine Science and the Cold War, 1946–65," *Southeast Asian Studies* 10, no. 1 (2021): 53–87; Vivek Neelakantan, "Disease Eradication and National Reconstruction," *IIAS Newsletter* 71 (2015): 4–5.

16 For understanding the historical context of regionalization, see Cueto, *The Value of Health.*
    Philip Havik and José Pedro Monteiro, "Portugal, the World Health Organization and the Regional Office for Africa: From Founding Member to Outcast," *The Journal of Imperial and Commonwealth History* 49, no. 4 (2021): 712–41. Havik and Monteiro's article discusses the evolution of regional bodies responsible for coordination of health in Africa. The authors depict how tensions between constructive international and regional engagement on the one hand and colonial sovereignty on the other played out and shifted in the African region.
    For the Southeast Asian context, see Monica Saavedra, "Politics and Health at the WHO Regional Office for Southeast Asia: The Case of Portuguese India, 1949–61," *Medical History* 61, no. 3 (2017): 380–400. Saavedra's research reveals how the 1950–61 conflict between Portugal and India over the territories that constituted Portuguese India, that is, Goa and Daman and Diu, informed Portugal's relations with the SEARO. The Goa question reveals the political production of the SEARO as a dynamic space for disputes between nation states in decolonizing Asia.

17 Sunil Amrith, *Decolonizing International Health: India and Southeast Asia, 1930–65* (Basingstoke: Palgrave Macmillan, 2006), 12–13.

18 Ibid.

19 Ibid., 13.

20 Ibid.

21 Incidentally Nationalist China was one of the sponsors of the San Francisco Conference. For details refer Szeming Sze, "Birth of the WHO: Interview with Szeming Sze," *World Health* (May 1989): 28–29, https://apps.who.int/iris/handle/10665/45224.

22 Szeming Sze, *The Origins of the World Health Organization: A Personal Memoir, 1945–48* (Boca Raton, FL: LISZ Publications, 1982).

23 "Discussion on the Report of the Interim Commission," Fifth Plenary Meeting, June 26, 1948, First World Health Assembly, *Official Records of the World Health Organization: Plenary Meetings, Main Committees and Summaries of*

Resolutions and Decisions No. 13 (Geneva: WHO, 1948), WHO Library and Historical Collections (WHOL).

24 Ibid.
25 See also Cueto, Brown and Fee, *The World Health Organization*, 63.
26 Ibid.
27 Cited in "Second World Health Assembly: Points from Speeches," *Chronicle of the World Health Organization* 3, no. 8 (1949): 220–21.
28 Amrith, *Decolonizing International Health*, 122.
29 Cueto, Brown and Fee, *The World Health Organization*, 64.
30 Ibid.
31 Ibid.
32 Ibid., 65.
33 Committee on Foreign Affairs, *Point Four: Background and Program* (Washington, DC: United States Government Printing Office, 1949), https://pdf.usaid.gov/pdf_docs/Pcaac280.pdf.
34 Maureen Gallagher, "The World Health Organization: Promotion of US and Soviet Policy Goals," *JAMA* 168, no. 1 (1963): 135–40
35 Gallagher, "The World Health Organization," 136.
36 Cueto, Brown and Fee, *The World Health Organization*, 66.
37 "Notification by the Union of Soviet Socialist Republics Concerning Participation in the World Health Organization," Executive Board Seventeenth Session Provisional Agenda Item 7.2, December 15, 1955, Doc. EB17/32, WHOL.
38 Cueto, Brown and Fee, *The World Health Organization*, 66.
39 Howard Calderwood, "The World Health Organization and Its Regional Organizations," *Temple Law Quarterly* 37, no. 1 (1963): 15–27.
40 Walter Sharp, "The New World Health Organisation," *American Journal of International Law* 41, no. 3 (1947): 509–30.
41 *Report of the Indian Delegation to the First Session of the World Health Assembly Held in Geneva from 24 June to 24 July 1948* (New Delhi: Government of India Press, 1948), 3.
42 Ibid.
43 Calderwood, "The World Health Organization," 18.
44 "Headquarters and Regional Organizations: Report by the Director General," Executive Board Second Session, August 27, 1948, Doc. EB2/24 (Geneva: WHO, 1948), WHOL.
45 "Rajkumari Amrit Kaur's Speech at the Fourth Plenary Meeting," Fourth Plenary Meeting, Second World Health Assembly, June 13–July 2, 1949, *Official Records of the World Health Organization: Second World Health Assembly Decisions and Resolutions* No. 21 (Geneva: WHO, 1949), WHOL.
46 "A Villarama at the Fifth Plenary Meeting," Fifth Plenary Meeting, Second World Health Assembly, June 13–July 2, 1949, *Official Records of the World Health Organization: Second World Health Assembly Decisions and Resolutions* No. 21 (Geneva: WHO, 1949), WHOL.
47 "A. Villarama at the Third Plenary Meeting," Third Plenary Meeting, Second World Health Assembly, June 13–July 2, 1949, *Official Records of the World Health Organization: Second World Health Assembly Decisions and Resolutions* No. 21 (Geneva: WHO, 1949), WHOL.
48 Martha May Eliot, "Report on Western Pacific," Committee on Programme (Seventeenth Meeting), Third World Health Assembly, May 8–27, 1950, *Official Records of the World Health Organization: Resolutions and Decisions, Plenary Meetings, Committees and Annexes* No. 28 (Geneva: WHO, 1950), WHOL.

49 Second World Health Assembly, "Rights and Obligations of Associate Members and Other Territories in Regional Organizations," Doc. WHA 2.103 (Geneva: WHO, 1949), WHOL, https://apps.who.int/iris/bitstream/handle/10665/86193/WHA2.103_eng.pdf;sequence=1.

50 Memorandum Issued by the Director General of Public Health, "Regarding the First WHO Meeting," May 11, 1948, *Algemeen Secretarie een de Daarbij Gedepoineerde Archiven (1942–50)*, Inventory Number 5102, Algemeen Rijksarchief (National Archives of the Netherlands or AR).

51 Memorandum Issued by the Lt. Governor General of the Netherlands Indies, "WHO Conferentie te Genève," June 14, 1948, *Algemeen Secretarie een de Daarbij Gedepoineerde Archiven (1942–50)*, Inventory Number 5102, AR. See also Neelakantan, *Science, Public Health and Nation-Building*, 68.

52 Third World Health Assembly, "Request by the Republic of the United States of Indonesia for Inclusion in the South-East Asia Area," Supplementary Agenda Item 13.2, May 12, 1950, Doc. A3/85, WHOL.

53 SEARO, *A Healthier Southeast Asia: 70 Years of WHO in the Region* (New Delhi: SEARO, 2018), 22.

54 Ibid., 23.

55 Twelfth World Health Assembly, "Participation of the Union of Soviet Socialist Republics in the Work of the Regional Committee for Southeast Asia," April 2, 1959, Provisional Agenda Item 7.11, Doc. A12/AFL/6, WHOL.

56 Calderwood, "The World Health Organization," 20.

57 Kelley Lee, *Historical Dictionary of the World Health Organization* (Lanham, MD: Scarecrow Press, 1998).

58 "C. Mani at the Third Meeting," Minutes of the Technical Preparatory Committee for the International Health Conference Held in Paris from March 18–April 5, 1946," *Official Records of the World Health Organization* No. 1 (UN, New York: WHO Interim Commission, 1946), WHOL.

59 World Health Organization, *Twenty Years in Southeast Asia, 1948–67* (New Delhi: SEARO, 1967), 66.

60 Ibid., 67.

61 Ibid.

62 Ibid.

63 SEARO Regional Committee, *Report of the Regional Director for 1949*, Third Session (Ceylon), September 22–26 1950, Doc. SEA/RC/3 (New Delhi: SEARO, 1950), WHOL.

64 "Letter from Cora Du Bois to C. Mani, Regional Director of the SEARO," June 6, 1950, Reports on the Field from Cora Dubois to SEARO: March–June 1950, Box 67, *Cora Du Bois Papers*, Box 67, Tozzer Library Special Collection, Harvard University.

65 Ibid.

66 Socrates Litsios, "Cora Du Bois Brief Stint with the World Health Organization (1950–51): Right Time, Wrong Place," *International Journal of Health Services* 48, no. 4 (2018): 716–34.

67 SEARO Regional Committee, *Third Annual Report of the Regional Director to the Regional Committee for Southeast Asia*, Fourth Session (Rangoon, Burma), September 20–25, 1951, Doc. SEA/R4/2 (New Delhi: SEARO, 1951), WHOL.

68 Ibid.

69 S.L. Dhir and A. Rahim, "Malaria Control in Afghanistan, 1950–54," *Indian Journal of Malariology* 11 (1957): 73–126.

70 "Letter from Robert Watson to Paul Russell, Malariologist," March 3, 1950, Folder 5188, Box 475, Series 100: Staff International, RG 2, Rockefeller Archive Center (RAC).

71 Ibid.
72 Ibid.
73 "Letter from C. Mani, Regional Director of the SEARO to Bonne," May 11, 1949, Southeast Asia: Program of Activities, Subject 902 Regional Organisations, Series 1, File 8, WHO *First and Second Generation Files*, WHOA.
74 World Health Organization, *Twenty Years*, 116.
75 Ibid., 117.
76 SEARO, *A Healthier Southeast Asia*, 27.
77 Chandra Mani, "International Health: Application of WHO Programs and Policies in a Region," *American Journal of Public Health* 41 (December 1951): 1469–72.
78 Mani, "International Health," 1470.
79 SEARO Regional Committee, "Proposed Program for Southeast Asia, 1951," June 30, 1950, Doc/RC3/1. Rev1, WHOL.
80 Niels Brimnes, *Languished Hopes: Tuberculosis, the State and International Assistance in Twentieth Century India* (Hyderabad: Orient BlackSwan, 2016), 114–15.
81 Ibid.
82 See also Vivek Neelakantan, "Tuberculosis Control in Postcolonial South India and Southeast Asia: Fractured Sovereignties in International Health, 1948–60," *Wellcome Open Research* 2, no. 4 (2018), https://doi.org/10.12688/wellcomeopenres.10544.2.
83 Brimnes, *Languished Hopes*, 135.
84 Ibid.
85 Vivek Neelakantan, "The Campaign Against the Big Four Endemic Diseases and Indonesia's Engagement with the Cold War, 1950s," in *Public Health and National Reconstruction in Cold War Asia: International Influences, Local Transformations*, edited by Liping Bu and Ka-che Yip (Abingdon, Oxon: Routledge, 2014), 154–74.
86 Government of India, *First Five Year Plan* (New Delhi: The Publications Division, Ministry of Information and Broadcasting, 1953), 21.
87 Tharaphi Than, "The Languages of Pyidawtha and the Burmese Approach to National Development," *Southeast Asia Research* 21, no. 4 (2013): 639–54.
88 SEARO, *Fifth Annual Report of the Regional Director to the Regional Committee for Southeast Asia: July 1952–July 1953*, July 1953, Doc. SEA/RC6/2 (New Delhi: SEARO, 1953), WHOL.
89 Ibid.
90 USPHS, *Joint Staff Conference: World Health Organization-Technical Cooperation Administration*, February 12–19, 1953 (Washington, DC: US Public Health Service).
91 Christopher Lee, "Final Communiqué of the Asian-African Conference," *Interventions: International Journal of Postcolonial Studies* 11, no. 1 (2009): 94–102.
92 Ibid., 101.
93 "Text of Address of Welcome by Dr Johannes Leimena, Minister of Health, Republic of Indonesia," *SEARO Regional Committee Eighth Session, Bandung*, September 5–10, 1955, Doc. SEA/RC8/Min.1/Rev.1, WHOL.
94 For a comprehensive understanding of the Mutual Security Administration refer "The Mutual Security Act of 1951," Public Law 165: 82nd Congress, Chapter 479 (1st Session), HR 5113, Longhand Notes Files, 1945–53, *President's Secretary Files: Truman Administration (1945–60)*, National Archives Identifier 28454324, National Archives and Records Administration (NARA), https://catalog.archives.gov/id/28454324.

95 Socrates Litsios, "Rural Hygiene in the Early Years of the World Health Organization: Another Casualty of the Cold War?", *Anais do Instituto de Higiene e Medicina Tropical* 16 (August 2016): 125–32.

96 Ibid., 131.

97 "Report on Development of Malaria Eradication Programme," May 4, 1959,Twelfth World Health Assembly, Provisional Agenda Item 6.5, Doc.A12/P&B/10, WHOL.

98 SEARO, *A Healthier Southeast Asia*, 35.

99 Neelakantan, "The Campaign Against the Big Four," 160.

100 Ibid., 162.

101 "Rural Health Conference, New Delhi (October 14–26, 1957)," Project SEARO 20 TA, *The Work of the WHO, 1957: Official Records of the World Health Organization* No. 82 (Geneva: WHO, 1957), WHOL.

102 The budgetary squeeze in Burma and Indonesia curtailed the malaria eradication program after 1958. Both nations also suffered threats to internal security. See for example, SEARO, *Report on the Thirteenth Session of the SEARO Held in Bandung, Indonesia (August 22–29, 1960)*, Doc. SEA/RC13/16 Rev.1 (New Delhi: SEARO, 1960), WHOL.

103 *Report on the Thirteenth Session of the SEARO.*

104 "Speech by President Soekarno to the Participants of the Southeast Asian Regional Conference of the WHO: Istana Bogor," August 28, 1960, *Pidato Presiden Republik Indonesia*, Arsip Nomor 209, Arsip Nasional Republik Indonesia (National Archives of Indonesia or ANRI).

105 Atsuko Naono, "'Rural' Health in Modern Southeast Asia," in *Histories of Health in Southeast Asia: Perspectives on the Long Twentieth Century*, edited by Tim Harper and Sunil Amrith (Bloomington: Indiana University Press, 2014), 99–117.

106 Amrith, *Decolonizing International Health*, 102.

107 Ibid.

108 Neelakantan, *Science, Public Health and Nation-Building*, 205–6.

2 The Cold War, Non-Alignment, and Medicine in India

The Case of Medical Education and Pharmaceutical Self-Sufficiency, 1947–57

Shirish Kavadi

Introduction

At the time of independence in 1947—as was the case with other newly independent states of Asia such as the Philippines, Indonesia, and Ceylon—the postcolonial state in India was faced with the challenge of transforming the society and economy along modern lines. In 1950, the Planning Commission was created with the then Prime Minister Jawaharlal Nehru as its first chairman. As a strong proponent of science and technology, Nehru was of the conviction that India needed to harness science for nation-building. To this end, the country needed to train a new generation of Indians who would apply science to solve national problems. In his mission to reconcile India's vision to contribute to international science and orient scientists to nation-building, Nehru was aided by the Indian colloid chemist Shanti Swarup Bhatnagar (also the founder of the Council of Scientific and Industrial Research or CSIR), Indian astrophysicist Meghnad Saha, and physicist Homi Bhabha. Bhabha laid the foundation for India's nuclear program. In the field of medicine, Nehru's efforts were driven by Amrit Kaur, India's first Minister of Health (1947–57).

Public health and scientific medicine had been internationalized in colonial India since the nineteenth century and also deeply contested.[1] It was further internationalized by the Rockefeller Foundation's public health programs beginning in 1920.[2] Medical education and research programs in the post-independence period simultaneously promoted and protected US interests in India in the context of the Cold War.[3] Foreign aid—influenced by the concerns of the Cold War, alongside domestic priorities—had a bearing on India's health and medical programs and policies. For instance, the engagement of the USSR in India's health sector was limited primarily to the manufacture of pharmaceuticals. It was part of the broader industrialization policy and hence it was handled not by the Health Ministry but by the Ministry of Commerce and Industry.[4]

The reorganization and transformation of India's public health and medical system was a nation-building project whose advancement was shaped by

DOI: 10.4324/9781003332060-3

the interface between international and domestic factors. The Indian national movement had advocated health as a civic right and state responsibility as well as an instrument for economic development.[5] By the eve of India's independence, the inadequacies of India's health and medical system were documented through reports from various committees, of which the Health Survey and Development Committee—constituted by the Government of India and chaired by Sir Joseph Bhore (the Bhore Committee)—for India's post-war reconstruction holds special significance. It was given the task of undertaking a survey of existing medical and health services and making recommendations for future planning of medical and healthcare in India. The Bhore Report (1946) noted a deficient medical infrastructure and scarcity of competently trained medical personnel, the consequences of which were limited, ineffective, and iniquitous access to proper health and medical care for the rural population in India.

The country's own approaches to health and medicine and the discourse on medical education specifically during this period were framed primarily around the recommendations of the Health Sub-Committee headed by Santok Singh Sokhey (Sokhey Committee, 1948) of the National Planning Committee (NPC) constituted by the Indian National Congress. The NPC, consisting of politicians, economists, scientists, and industrialists, stood for state planning, industrialization, and community development.

The chapter examines the various debates, developments, and attempts to reform medical development in the early years after independence, with a special focus on medical education and the development of the pharmaceutical industry, in two sections. These are examined in the context of India's endeavors toward development, modernization, and nation-building, and the rivalry between the US and the USSR during the Cold War (1950s), as the domestic and the international were closely intertwined and had a bearing on the health and medical fields. The initial framing of medical education policies during the tenure of Rajkumari Amrit Kaur, the first Cabinet Health Minister in the National Government from 1947 to 1957, and as discussed and critiqued by scholars, is examined.[6]

The public discourse since independence primarily concerned quantity versus quality. Some stressed the former, pointing to the USSR and how it had, through short-term courses, turned out doctors in quantity as if through a mill. Those who considered the shortage of personnel as the "real bottleneck" argued that India should emulate other countries such as the Soviet Union and "put into motion the Man-Making Machine" to turn out the necessary numbers. It was pointed out that the Soviet Union after the 1917 revolution had successfully augmented the number of doctors by enlarging the number of student admissions in existing institutions and training them through a shift system commonly practiced in factories. Soviet determination had seen its doctor strength enhanced fivefold in 15 years. If India were to show similar resolve, it could achieve this goal in 25 years.[7] Others differed with critics, considering these steps to introduce short-term courses for producing doctors to be retrogressive, cheap, easy, and haphazard, which would only produce "raw and callow half-baked medical practitioners" and would "bring down deliberately the standard of medical qualifications even lower than what it was previously."[8]

Amrit Kaur looked to the West and sought assistance—particularly from the US—for her plans for medical education in India whereas Sokhey sought to build self-sufficiency in the Indian pharmaceutical industry from scratch with the assistance of the USSR. The two case studies related to Indian medical education and pharmaceutical self-sufficiency provide a unique opportunity for historians to examine one of the most pressing questions concerning international health today—the implementation of aid during the early Cold War. At the time, India tried to achieve a delicate balance between self-sufficiency and increased openness to international aid. Questions broached by the chapter include: (a) What was the nature of the influence of the USA and the USSR on medical projects supported by them during this period? (b) What kind of medical programs were they involved with? (c) What is the relationship between those who give aid and those who receive it?

Nehruvian Science and Nation-Building

Much has been written about Nehru's intense personal and philosophical fervor for science and his advocacy for science and technology in building the new nation.[9] This partly arose from his conviction that both the US and the USSR achieved rapid development using science and technology. Nehru hoped not only to tailor scientific research to Indian problems but also to train a new generation of Indians in research skills and inculcate scientific temper.[10] He held the portfolio of Scientific Research and his Government prioritized and vigorously pursued scientific research and technical education, leading to the establishment of five Indian Institutes of Technology (IITs) and the All India Institute of Medical Sciences (AIIMS).

In Nehru's conviction, science and technology constituted a "state science" and a national "institution-building project."[11] Scientific research was to be conducted at the state's direction and discretion. Nehru's vision was shared and supported by India's protagonists of national science, including Saha, Bhaba, and Santok Singh Sokhey. Some of these scientists such as Saha and Sokhey were close to the Communist Party of India. Their engagement with Indian science coincided with the notorious McCarthy Era and hence the Americans were somewhat suspicious of them.[12] It must also be noted that Sokhey was a confirmed radical with leftist leanings who did not conceal his ideological sympathies. In 1947, he was awarded the Lenin Peace Prize at a time when Indo-USSR relations were not very close. He visited China after the communist takeover and returned much impressed.[13] Sokhey was elected President of the All-India Peace Council, a part of the World Peace Council, and later on, the President of the

Association of Scientific Workers of India (ASWI), the Indian branch of the World Federation of Scientific Workers. Nehru was the first president of the ASWI in 1947.[14]

Saha, apart from his involvement with science, was attracted towards planning and the socialist experiment in the Soviet Union. Saha persuaded Subhash Chandra Bose, as the President of the Indian National Congress, to set up a Planning Committee which was headed by Nehru.[15] There is an aspect of planning that needs to be noted for it reflected how India attempted to navigate the Cold War and express its non-aligned stance. In the words of Nikhil Menon:

> "an arranged marriage between Soviet – inspired economic planning and Western-style liberal democracy, at a time when the Cold War portrayed them as ideologically contradictory and institutionally incompatible......economic planning in India was considerably different from the kind practiced in communist regimes. The Planning Commission was reined in by democratic procedure that required consultation with ministries in an elected government, with people's representatives in Parliament-and ultimately with the popular will-through citizens voting every five years."[16]

The expansion of CSIR laboratories and the IITs was an outcome of this vision of planning and the importance of science for a self-reliant India. Nehru's scientist colleagues used their international network to develop India's scientific and technological program.[17]

Negotiating the Cold War and Development Politics in India, 1947–57

Three major developments that reshaped the international order in the mid-twentieth century included World War II, decolonization, beginning with Indonesia (1945), the Philippines (1946), and India consecutively, and the onset of the Cold War between the US and the USSR. International health, in turn, was informed by these events. In its bid to buttress Asia against communist ideology, the US, under the Truman and Eisenhower administrations, adopted a comprehensive program of technical assistance for newly independent nations, often in the form of humanitarian assistance. The rationale for this was straightforward: poverty was the breeding ground of communism. Since disease caused poverty, eradicating disease would prevent the spread of communism to developing countries. The articulation of international development, particularly during the early 1950s, coincided with US national interests that sought to increase the flow of raw materials from developing countries to industrial centers and provide overseas markets for US goods.[18] In the 1950s' Cold War context, India sought to maintain a delicate balance between increased openness to overseas technical assistance and self-sufficiency.

The aid relationships that developed between the US, international organizations, and the newly independent nations during the 1950s have been characterized by David Engerman as "development politics."[19] He states that these relationships "relied upon tight connections between the US, international aid agencies and individual ministries." During the 1950s, development politics was autonomous of the central decision-making bodies of newly independent countries.

With the emerging Cold War, many newly independent countries led by India, Indonesia, and Burma disembarked on a policy of non-alignment by refusing to get entangled in a rivalry they considered essentially European. The Indian Government sought to balance the influence of the two blocs since it was aware that it needed assistance from both sides and from international organizations. As Manu Bhagavan comments, "Indian foreign and domestic policy in this context was broadly concerned with great power politics, peacemaking, and economic development."[20] For instance, India's intercession between the two Super Powers and advances toward the USSR had in fact started during the early 1950s with the outbreak of the Korean War. In other words, India's intercession in Korea embodied the principle of non-alignment.

By 1949, China engaged in a civil war and fell to the Communists. India—given its strategic location, enormous population, and the political aspirations of Nehru in freeing India from either Soviet or American affiliations—became central to the Cold War.[21] Both the Soviets and the Americans were of the conviction that if they could influence the mode of economic and social development in India, the country could serve as a model for other new nations in Asia and Africa. India in turn, with its policy of non-alignment and a mixed economy, hoped to derive political capital from the Cold War politics in Asia and sought to receive technical aid from both the US and the USSR for nation-building.

Rajkumari Amrit Kaur as Health Minister

One of the specific recommendations the Bhore Committee made was the creation of a Central Ministry of Health for India. Amrit Kaur's name was proposed as Minister in the interim Government in 1946 but was turned down by Viceroy Mountbatten.[22] When the first Cabinet was sworn in on August 15, 1947, Nehru appointed her as independent India's first Union Cabinet Health Minister—an office that she held until April 1957. Born into the royal family of Patiala and Christian by confession, educated in the UK, an excellent tennis player, inspired by Gandhian ideology, committed to the betterment of women and children and active participation in international aid agencies sums up her personality. Amrit Kaur was a member of the Lok Sabha (lower chamber of the Indian Parliament) and Rajya Sabha between

1952 and 1962, respectively. She represented India at the World Health Assembly and International Red Cross. She introduced family planning in India while emphasizing the Gandhian approach of abstinence.[23]

Recently, scholars have examined Amrit Kaur's role in spearheading the cause for political participation of women. Amrit Kaur was an early leader of several important women's organizations in India. These included the All-India Women's Conference (AIWC) and the Young Women's Christian Association-India (YWCA India). This enabled her to serve as the liaison to Western-dominated international women's organizations such as the International Council of Women (ICW). Emily Rook-Koepsel observes, "Today, Amrit Kaur has become a footnote in the history of India's independence and its women's movement; she comes up periodically as the first woman government minister, as a confidant of Gandhi, or as leader of the early women's movement."[24] Her conception of locally engaged work as a foundation for citizenship and her eschewing of the state as the sole guarantor of citizenship rights, however, have continued to be aspirational for women's activism and in critiques of the state in India. Her association with these international associations gave her the international recognition, connections, and access to other international organizations and foreign governments that she would approach in later years.

There are a few articles in popular and official publications paying tributes to her and passing references to her in memoirs and literature on health and medicine. [25] Accounts about AIIMS make only laudatory references to Amrit Kaur but there is no detailed study of her role and contribution to her other wide-ranging efforts to develop medical education or infrastructure.[26]

While her personality and character evoked respect, she does not appear to have been proportionately influential within domestic politics. It may not be incorrect to observe that she was politically ineffectual. She was a member of the Indian Parliament from independence up to her death in 1962. She was denied a ticket to contest the 1957 Lok Sabha elections and instead compensated with an elevation to the Rajya Sabha. She lost her ministerial post that was instead given to D P Karmarkar, a Minister of State who had previously held the post in the Commerce Ministry. Karmarkar appears to have had little interest in Health.[27] Amrit Kaur was placated with the Chairperson's office of the Governing Board of the AIIMS. All of this indicates respect but simultaneously underscores her position as a political lightweight. This maybe a partial explanation why most historical accounts of health policy, public health, and medical care in post-independent India have paid little attention to Amrit Kaur as India's first Minister of Health and her contribution to developing medical science in the early years of India's independence.[28]

Among Kaur's closest supporters were Dr. Jivraj Mehta, a Bombay doctor and nationalist, who held the posts of both Health Secretary and Director General of Health Services for a brief period; K.C.K.E. Raja from the All India Institute of Hygiene and Public Health (AIIHPH) who later became of DGHS; and Dr. C.G. Pandit, Secretary of the Indian Council of Medical Research (ICMR) and a former Rockefeller fellow in whom she had "an abiding faith." Other supporters of Amrit Kaur included Dr. V.R. Khanolkar, Director of the Indian Cancer Research Center (ICRC) and India's leading medical and cancer researcher at the time; and B.B. Dikshit, the first Director of AIIMS. On the contrary, none of the scientists close to Nehru's inner circle supported her initiatives. The Medical Council of India maintained an antagonistic attitude toward the Ministry of Health over the question of medical education.[29]

Amrit Kaur attempted to locate her own medical projects within Nehruvian science, as seen in the zeal she displayed in establishing the AIIMS (modeled on the lines of Johns Hopkins Medical School). To realize her institute-building project for public health in postcolonial India—particularly pertaining to the training of medical professionals overseas and the construction of the ICMR building and the National Medical Library—she liaised with US philanthropic foundations (such as the Rockefellers), the WHO, and UNICEF.[30] AIIMS was among a series of science laboratories and technology institutes established during the Nehruvian Era, fitting within his vision for India's development and nation-building efforts, but it was Amrit Kaur who was the driving force behind it.

The efforts of Amrit Kaur were directed at: (a) reforming the colonial organization of medical research; and (b) institutionalization of medical research that was at once relevant to India's immediate needs and the world of science. While Amrit Kaur's efforts were visionary, the implementation was flawed. For example, there was a clear inconsistency in policies such as sending students abroad for study and expecting them to work on India-related problems but with no assurance of a job on return considering the kind of training they had received abroad. Her commitment to health and medicine also displayed the same centralizing tendencies that were a crucial feature of Nehru toward planning, development, and modernization. Her overwhelming zeal led state governments to express fear that medical education, which was a state subject, was being increasingly centralized—but she also appeared to be constrained by the priorities of the wider planning process and her limited political influence.[31]

Technical Assistance from the WHO, USAID, and the Rockefeller Foundation to India

Historically, for a brief phase after the end of the Second World War, the USSR was not a part of international organizations such as the WHO, which in the delivery of its services and in providing aid for development activities, had to deal with Cold War politics. Due to its ideological differences with the US over socialized medicine, the USSR, from 1948 to 1956, stayed out of the WHO. As Elizabeth Fee, Theodore Brown, and Marcos Cueto observe, "The Organization became captive of US political interests, embarked on a limited program of disease control, and settled upon an institutional structure of regionalization."[32] This partly explains why the USSR had no direct engagement with the Ministry of Health or the ICMR in the development of India's health and medical programs.

On the contrary, in the American case, John A. Logan argued to the effect that the US needed to use foreign assistance programs to counteract Communism, stating "our interests are ultimately and irrevocably linked with all of the other countries on the globe. The success or failure of our Technical and Foreign Aid program is, therefore, of very real importance. Public health workers, who have served for more than a century as a 'social conscience' with regard to the improvement of health and sanitation in the US, must now apply the same approach to the world. In helping to raise social and economic standards in the underdeveloped areas, public health can be used to combat communism at its most vulnerable point."[33] Consequently, the WHO and the UNICEF became prisoners of US foreign policy.

As newly independent India embarked on a program of nation building, the government undertook a program of knowledge production and international exchange referred to as "brain irrigation," which involved opening up opportunities for knowledge exchange between Indian scientists and foreign experts.[34] Apart from the government-to-government contacts, this opened up opportunities for foreign foundations. Leonard Gordon calls the 1950s and the 1960s "the golden age of the big foundations in India."[35]

The United States was a major donor to India, providing technical assistance for health and sanitation amounting to $107 million from 1950 to 1973.[36] Roger Jeffery notes that there was "something of a division of labor between US aid and that of the WHO." US aid provided for material supplies while technical advisers, many of them American, were sent by the WHO which, as explained earlier, was virtually dominated by American experts. Indians were also trained in the US, for example, between 1952 and 1960, 249 Indians were trained in health subjects.[37] The UNICEF, often along with WHO, provided substantial assistance to health programs especially related to maternal and child health service, disease control programs such as tuberculosis (TB) and leprosy, the manufacture of vaccines, and to the applied nutrition program. From 1947 to 1970, the UNICEF contributed US$64 million, mostly demarcated for the implementation of India's public health programs.[38] The WHO was also a generous donor, with over $40 million provided from 1948 to the mid-1970s.[39] As was the case with US aid, the monetary support from WHO was substantially distributed to the Government's communicable disease control and eradication program that included malaria, smallpox, and tuberculosis, part of which went to technical advisers and fellowships for Indians to study abroad. WHO was also a source of both formal and informal technical assistance.

The WHO, along with USAID, Ford, and Rockefeller advisers, attended and sometimes contributed to meetings of the Central Council of Health during the 1950s and early 1960s.[40] These advisers evaluated plans and projects. Their support, Jeffery notes, was crucial to the disease control programs, especially malaria, during this period.[41] The "non-political" status of these international organizations placed them in an advantageous position vis-a-vis Americans. The advice from WHO and UNICEF made US technical assistance more palatable to newly decolonized countries of Asia and Africa during the 1950s.[42] But as stated above, in practice the philanthropic organizations worked closely with USAID at the peak of their assistance during this period.[43] Until the 1960s, American aid accounted for a substantial part of India's technical assistance in health.

Rajkumari Amrit Kaur, the Rockefeller Foundation, and Medical Education in India

At independence, India had approximately 50,000 doctors and a doctor–patient ratio of approximately 1–per 7000. Among the immediate measures undertaken by the Government of India to address this deficit of physicians were: 1) the elevation of medical schools to medical colleges; 2) the abolition of the licentiate diploma; 3) upgrading of particular departments or sections in select existing medical colleges and institutions to postgraduate training and research facilities; and 4) the establishment of new medical colleges in different parts of the country. The last step saw the number of new medical colleges increase from 14 to 24 between 1947 and 1952.[44] During the First Five-Year Plan the number went up from 30 to 42 and the number of student admissions from 2,500 in 1950–51 to 3,500 in 1957 when the second general elections were held and Amrit Kaur dropped as the Health Minister.[45] As pointed out, early funding of the Health Ministry programs was inadequate and this expansion could barely be expected to meet India's needs. Tensions over finances between the Health Ministry and the Ministry of Finance and the Planning Commission were not uncommon but there were other problems that had more serious ramifications for medical education and personnel policy as well, discussed below.

The Health Ministry received its first setback when its budget for 1949–50 was "cut down absolutely to the bone."[46] Amrit Kaur informed the press that her Ministry had contemplated an expenditure of about Rs. 4.5 million on the capital side but it was halved to a mere Rs. 2 million. On the revenue side, it was reduced to Rs. 10 million from the proposed Rs. 20 million. These cuts would adversely affect plans for rural health centers and hospital expansion, and delay the founding of the All India Medical Institute, apart from cancelation of the five overseas scholarships budgeted for.[47] However, Amrit Kaur's regular public expression of her grievances incurred Nehru's disapproval, who considered it improper for a minister. Nehru wrote: "Sometimes in your earnestness and enthusiasm for improving the Health Services of the nation, you condemn the Government of India generally and more particularly the Finance Ministry for not providing enough funds." The government's allocation of funds was ultimately "determined by some planned approach to the various problems of India." Progress of all sectors was essential and health services would be "absolutely useless" if there was not enough food available in the country, which was "the primary factor for health." No services would function adequately, Nehru asserted, "if there is anarchy in the country."[48] Nehru's letter to Kaur highlights the government's prioritization of industrialization.

The ICMR derived all its funds from the Central Government. Provincial governments paid little contribution despite appeals. The ICMR was financially constrained. In 1947 its grants from the government were barely Rs. 1.2 million a year and rose to a mere Rs. 5 million in 1964. In real terms this was not clearly much of an improvement.[49] Appeals to the states to allocate separate funds for research had no effect. As the Health Ministry began to roll out its plans for medical education and research, it turned to the Rockefeller Foundation—not only for technical expertise but also for financial aid, a carry-over of the approach from the interwar years and common to the Rockefeller Foundation's global experience.

The Second Five-Year Plan was expected to make available larger allocations to research in comparison to the previous one. However, there were others who were not confident about these developments. Dr. C.S. Thakar, a prominent medical practitioner and office bearer in the Indian Medical Association, delivering the Presidential Address at the All-India Medical Conference in February 1957 stressing the importance of creating a research environment, establishing of facilities, and creating opportunities in medical research, considered the provision of Rs. 40 million made in the plan as "grossly inadequate" and observed that, "Research is a necessary adjunct to the practice of modern scientific medicine and needs to be freely encouraged with ample funds."[50] Several international and multilateral organizations had been extending aid for equipment for various scientific and other purposes. But a shortfall in the Plan funds and a shortage of foreign exchange caused by heavy imports in the initial years of independence upset much of the Plan goals. This had an adverse bearing on research activities in India. The Indian government, in order to conserve foreign currency, placed restrictions on imports, permitting only those that were directly related to economic development.

In August 1957, a deputation of the Indian Medical Association met with Nehru and complained about the curbs on import of medical equipment. Nehru wrote to Finance Minister T. T. Krishnamachari, reminding him that he "disliked the idea of discouraging research." He believed that doctors should be encouraged to possess "their tools of trade and profession" and the government "should encourage initiative and love of research and the building up of laboratories."[51] Nehru's intervention did not help much. Krishnamachari resigned and Morarji Desai, elected to the Parliament from Bombay Province and a cabinet minister, was put in charge in March 1958. Under Desai, foreign aid and imports of medical research equipment continued to be restricted.

Literature on the history of health and medicine after independence has characterized health and medical planning as state-directed and centralized, with disease control programs having a sturdy techno-managerial orientation. Historians have referred to the paradoxes and contradictions that featured prominently in planning, policies, and programs affecting adversely the development of India's medical and health system. They note a paradox in India: a strong interventionist state committed to welfare and development which, however, did not prioritize health in planning.[52]

During the 1950s, Indian authorities pursued two contradictory goals in medical education: (a) modernizing to attain western standards in medical education and research; and (b) seeking to ensure that it was relevant to India's needs. In the conflict between the two, modernization of medical education overrode the goal of seeking to make medical education relevant to India's needs.[53] Several of India's prominent medical professionals and leaders, both during the colonial period and after independence, were trained in modern medicine by acquiring post-graduate education abroad. On their return, their efforts were directed at "keeping up with the West."

The Rockefeller Fellowship Program and Nehru's Reservations of US Technical Assistance

Noting that the Rockefeller Foundation's traditional public health and disease control programs were in danger of being overshadowed by those of the WHO and the Pan-American Sanitary Bureau, Rockefeller's officials suggested a re-orientation in its approach.[54] In 1944, John Grant, the Director of the All India Institute for Hygiene and Public Health between 1939 and 1945, explicated the need for a post-war health policy for India. Such a policy would help the local governments to implement their own medical programs. In India, he noted, the chief obstacle was the lack of personnel, both in numbers and in specialization.[55] In 1948, the WHO instituted nursing and research fellowships to young medical researchers to pursue postgraduate degrees. In 1948, Amrit Kaur approached the Foundation to support a fellowship program, renewed every 3 years, which came to an end in 1961. The candidates were selected and recommended by the Central Health Ministry through a committee appointed for the purpose, which caused much resentment among state governments.[56]

Grant, while still Director of the All India Institute of Hygiene and Public Health, had recommended a personnel training program that had to be "self-contained" for, he observed, "There is not much real lasting value until a country can train its own teachers."[57] On the contrary, the Vice President of the Rockefeller Foundation, Alan Gregg, suggested "We can, with real elegance, back the good men who are in India, and we can find the good men who are in India, through our fellowship program, and then back them up when they come back. Backing good Indians who are now there and backing others, now and in the future, would give competent men to India."[58]

Foreign fellowships and travel grants were intended to give the training and experience in the US to junior medical faculty that was unobtainable in India. The duration of fellowships covered instruction in comprehensive medical care and nursing, and were broad-based to include both basic sciences and clinical subjects. College authorities were required to give an assurance that the teachers, on their return, would be given opportunities to conduct research in their specialized areas.

However, even as the Government of India negotiated with the US agencies and the Rockefeller Foundation, there were reservations about the international exchange program. Nehru expressed his discomfort with sending Indians abroad for training, and specifically about American aid, activities, attitudes, and visits of American experts, as some tended to give the impression of taking responsibility for government tasks which he viewed as interference in Indian affairs.[59] Nehru additionally deemed it undesirable for Indians to go to the US for training.[60] Saha, now a Member of Parliament, demanded that India revise and perfect its strategy of international scientific collaboration to ensure the country's eventual "technical autonomy"[61] while Mudaliar opposed sending doctors abroad for training, arguing India was self-sufficient.[62] Underlying Nehru's reticence to Rockefeller aid were the American criticism of his foreign policy, an attack on his person by resident American diplomats, and the US decision to extend military aid to Pakistan in 1954.[63]

In May 1953, Nehru wrote to C.D. Deshmukh, the then Finance Minister, that he disliked US government representatives having direct dealing with educational institutions, and expected funds to be distributed through the ministries concerned; he stressed that there was a need for prior approval from the Government of India, a check on American activities in India, and restrictions on exchange of persons between the two countries.[64] Harry Friedgood, Professor of Clinical Medicine, University of California, noted that cooperation between TCA or Technical Cooperation Administration—founded in 1950 by the Truman Administration to administer the Point Four Program of Technical Assistance—and the Health Ministry, was on a "must" basis, and "Indians don't relish it." The Finance Ministry considered it inexpedient to accept money from the US State Department.[65]

In December 1956, the Indian government forbade educational institutions from directly approaching any foreign government or agency for aid and assistance.[66] Amrit Kaur, who had established a rapport with the Rockefeller Foundation, had returned from a Foundation-guided visit to US medical institutes—including a meeting with Dean Rusk, US Assistant of State for East Asian and Pacific Affairs. In July 1956, Amrit Kaur requested technical assistance for several of her medical projects, including the AIIMS.[67] But she expected the Foundation's representatives to keep her ministry informed of any aid to the country's medical institutes to ensure it was in accordance with her ministry's plans and policies and to avoid duplication while preparing the country's Five-Year Plan.[68] From 1956, the

Foundation's officers were engaged in extensive negotiations with Indian officials, with little effect. By 1961, Indian educational institutions were further restrained from receiving direct foreign aid.

Amrit Kaur, the AIIMS, and Openness to Western Technical Assistance

Amrit Kaur's tenure would be primarily remembered for her enthusiastic and zealous pursuit of the founding of the All India Institute of Medical Sciences (AIIMS) in New Delhi. Modeled on the Johns Hopkins Medical School, it became India's premier medical institute. The establishment of AIIMS was part of Amrit Kaur's broader attempts and the culmination of the various measures she undertook for the professionalization and institutionalization of medical education and research in India that included: (a) seeking aid and assistance to promote fellowships for medical personnel in India and abroad; and (b) getting funds for construction of the ICMR building and the National Medical Library from international organizations—particularly the WHO, UNICEF, the Colombo Plan, and the Rockefeller Foundation. At a time when the Ministry of Finance showed a parsimonious attitude toward health and medicine, she managed to raise funds from international and foreign philanthropic agencies.

In 1952, Amrit Kaur approached Alan Gregg for support for the AIIMS from the Rockefeller Foundation but Gregg was reluctant to go ahead with the project which he said should not be undertaken before 1960. He felt that at that juncture it appeared inappropriate for the institute to become the primary claim on the Central Government. He also thought locating it in the capital would lead to jealousies and politics with state governments responsible for medical education resenting the national government supporting an All India Institute when it should be offering assistance to the states instead of shaming them. Also, there was the question as to whether it was practical to have just one more college when most colleges in the states were languishing for funds and personnel. He also raised issues regarding salaries for such an elite institution and the source of funding.[69]

Amrit Kaur went on to argue, "But what worries me is the fact that you consider the enterprise of the All India Medical Institute (AIMI) an unwise one. I myself am so anxious to raise standards of medical education in our country and to give our young men and women a chance of post-graduate studies in their own country and in their own rural background. Unless I have an institution under the Central Ministry of Health, I cannot achieve my object and therefore it is that I am trying to lay the foundation of what should be an ideal teaching institution in our country. Were our States not autonomous in the matter of Health I might have tried other ways and means of raising standards, as for example, by upgrading various departments or even upgrading standards in the existing colleges in India. That, however, is not possible for me to do with the present set-up. I believe that if the AIMI is started on a sound foundation it will eventually become not only a good centre for all the Indian States to copy but also an international centre for the South East Asia Zone."[70]

The decision to establish the institute had been made much earlier by the government and a staff recruitment and building program had been initiated, but negligible to limited provisions were made in the budget for the scheme. Annoyed with the attitude of the Ministry of Finance, she approached the Colombo Plan.[71] She managed to secure a generous contribution of $2 million from the New Zealand Government for AIIMS.[72] The AIIMS Bill Act was introduced in Parliament in February 1956. It was a comprehensive charter. While introducing the Bill, she repeated the arguments she had made to Gregg in her letter of June 1953 and stated that what was unique about the institute was that it was to be granted University status and that students passing out spread throughout the country to take up the training of medical personnel.[73] Once established, the Rockefeller Foundation granted the AIIMS over $1.2 million in assistance, and for its rural training center at Ballabgarh near Delhi over $250,000.[74]

The Rockefeller Foundation also established the Virus Research Centre (the present-day National Institute of Hygiene) in Poona and from 1950 to 1973 provided it major grants amounting to over $1.2 million. It also provided funding and aided selected medical colleges like the CMC Vellore, the Trivandrum Medical College, and the King George's Medical College, Lucknow, to set up Preventive and Social Medicine departments.[75] In 1955, it had sponsored national-level Medical Conferences in Bangalore and Bombay to discuss the introduction of Preventive and Social Medicine in medical colleges.[76]

Sokhey, USSR Technical Assistance, and the Quest for Pharmaceutical Self-Sufficiency

As explained earlier in the introduction, the USSR, until 1953, had limited engagement with India. Scholars such as Vijay Singh and Swapna Nayudu have discussed in detail Nehru's approach and dealings with the communists in India, his suspicions about them and his reservations about the Soviet leadership—especially Stalin—although there was a thaw under Nikita Khrushchev.[77]

Stalin died in March 1953, which caused much internal upheaval in the USSR. A process of de-Stalinization followed in the USSR under Nikita Khrushchev and N.A. Bulganin, and the former inaugurated the USSR's Peace Offensive.[78] The period that followed witnessed the internationalization of Soviet foreign policy that now extended well beyond the Socialist Bloc. There was particular emphasis on peaceful coexistence with the US that was broadened to include developing countries. India attracted Soviet aid after the Asian-African Conference at Bandung.[79]

After the demise of Stalin, as bilateral relations with the USSR improved, India felt increasingly confident about its new role in world politics. The USSR and India attended the Geneva Conference (1954) although the latter was uninvited. As a part of the agreement, the French agreed to withdraw their troops from northern Vietnam. The agreement at Geneva demonstrated that lasting peace could be achieved through diplomacy. Nehru suggested a six-point plan that included: (a) the promotion of a climate of peace and negotiation for the realization of which he appealed to all concerned to discard threats; (b) ceasefire in Indochina; (c) granting of independence to the Indochina states by France; (d) direct negotiations between the actual belligerents Ho Chi Minh and Bao Dai; (e) bringing about a solemn agreement among the US, the USSR, the UK, and the People's Republic of China; and seeking the UN's good offices for purposes of conciliation.[80] The Conference failed due to mutual suspicions between the West and China. At the Conference, the then Indian Defense Minister V.K. Krishna Menon liaised not with not only the Vietminh, China, and the USSR but also the French and the British in working out a neutralization formula that intended to preserve the sovereignty and territorial integrity of the Indochinese states.

In 1955, leaders of India and the USSR conducted bilateral visits. These visits laid the foundation for future technical collaborations. At the Asian-African Conference held at Bandung in 1955, Nehru emphasized "peaceful coexistence, keeping out of the two camps, and the social and economic progress of the newly decolonized countries."[81] The USSR viewed this as a positive sign on the part of India. Referring to these developments Manu Bhagavan observes, "Nikita Khrushchev's assumption of power afforded new possibilities and channels of communication, and a burst of sunshine amid otherwise gloomy forecasts. Nehru really believed that a turning point had been reached, or at least was near, not just in terms of bilateral relations, but in broader Cold War terms as well."[82] Nayudu notesthat the Soviet premier Georgy Malenkov was keen on communist-capitalist coexistence, in synchrony with India's broad vision for the world. At the same time, the Soviets saw support for decolonization as a means to draw newly forming nation-states into their sphere of influence.

Andreas Hilger points out that Soviet political aims in India were hindered by weaknesses and inner contradictions of the Soviet programs.[83] One instance may be cited here. The Soviet aid to establish the Indian Institute of Technology (IIT) Bombay from 1955 onwards ran into difficulties since the Soviets found that as per the original agreement, they were unable to provide enough English-speaking faculty and the IIT ironically had to rely predominantly on American and a few European teaching staff. Indian incorporation of the Soviet education model was selective, with the country prioritizing its own objectives. According to Hilger, "Indian development plans and ideas proved to have a decisive impact on the implementation of

Soviet initiatives and did not fit into the conventional pattern of the East-west conflict."[84]

The USSR provided scholarships for Indian students, but according to one source, only three students undertook higher education during the 1950s, whereas a few thousand Indian students undertook professional training in the US.[85] Part of the problem could be attributed to the USSR government's policy of discouraging the development of social engagements between Soviet citizens and foreigners, either abroad or in the Soviet Union. Education of Indian students at Soviet universities constituted only a limited contribution to the formation of Indian elites as these students, upon their return, for the lack of any kind of a network, were unable to influence institutional structure or policies.

Although India had a fledgling pharmaceutical sector in 1947, scientific research was absent, which hindered its growth, and made it difficult to address "the legal monopoly that the British-era Indian Patent Law provided to the multinationals."[86] Purkayastha observes, "This was a two-pronged battle, a battle to change the patent laws to serve the interests of the Indian people; the other, building the scientific infrastructure and know-how required by the indigenous drug industry."[87] In this situation, the cost of drugs in India was unaffordable to the large population still living in poverty with limited access to medical care. Recognizing this, the Indian Government decided it had to prioritize decreasing the prices of drugs and pharmaceuticals. The matter had received some attention even before independence. In 1945, the government of British India constituted a panel headed by R N Chopra to examine the issue. The objective was to make India self-reliant in fine chemicals, drugs, and pharmaceuticals within a decade-and-a-half.[88] Nehru's view of technological self-sufficiency was not shared by all cabinet ministers and the Medical Council of India.

The Government of India began to explore the possibilities of manufacturing pharmaceutical products specifically focusing on those required to prevent and treat communicable diseases, which were accorded the highest public health priority in India and other newly independent countries at the time. Between 1946 and 1948, technical teams visited pharmaceutical companies in Western Europe and North America to investigate chances for cooperation and collaboration in the manufacture of various drugs. Penicillin was of particular concern. The teams prioritized the production of penicillin, paludrine, and sulfa drugs in their proposal. In January 1949, the Government examined the proposal and chose to set up a corporation in the public sector to manufacture these pharmaceutical products.[89] Dominique A Tobbell has demonstrated how pharmaceutical companies—in their domestic struggle with the government—decided on the pricing of drugs and harnessed the Cold War to their advantage.[90] American companies appeared to be unlikely collaborators at a time when India was directing its efforts to reduce drug prices to make them affordable.

The person who played a significant part in developing India's capacities and self-sufficiency in drugs and pharmaceuticals was Santok Singh Sokhey. Sokhey was a member of the elite colonial Indian Medical Service and had been amongst the first batch of Indians as Rockefeller Foundation fellows. Sokhey was the first Indian to become the Director of the Haffkine Institute in Bombay which was primarily involved in research and manufacture of vaccines. Sokhey used his international connections in building the pharmaceutical and drug industry within the broader context of industrialization, import substitution policy, and self-reliance. Sokhey laid the blueprint for public-sector drug production.

Sokhey had begun to seriously contemplate and form views on the issue of drug production which he publicly articulated as early as 1942 at the Second Indian Pharmaceutical Conference. He declared that sufficiency of production of drugs in India itself was absolutely essential. In 1943, he visited Western Europe, the US, and Canada to understand their experience in this field.[91] The sector was dominated by large private corporations who were willing, under certain conditions, to undertake production in India. Between 1949 and 1952—subsequent to serving in the WHO for 3 years as Assistant Director of Technical Services with the responsibility for epidemiology, health statistics, and biological standardization—Sokhey returned to India in 1952. He facilitated the government's efforts in the establishment of Hindustan Antibiotics for the production of penicillin at Pimpri near Poona (Pune) and the establishment of a DDT factory with help of the WHO and UNICEF.[92]

Between 1953 and 1958, with a view to ensuring the country's self-sufficiency in the production of essential drugs, the Indian government was faced with two policy choices: (a) sponsoring a fully integrated state-owned complex of pharmaceutical plants supported by the USSR; or (b) reliance on US and West German technical knowhow and financial investments for both state-owned and privately owned pharmaceutical companies.[93] India's Second Five-Year Plan (1956–61) emphasized building the country's capacity in the production of heavy organic chemicals, pharmaceutical intermediaries, and bulk drug capacities. During the formulation of India's Second Five-Year Plan, the Planning Commission's advocacy for involving the private sector in drug development drew Nehru's attention. He made the categorical point that the base of the pharmaceutical industry should lie in the public sector, although influential members in the cabinet such as T.T. Krishnamachari opposed Nehru's views.[94] Indian industrialists did not favor Nehru's advocacy for development of India's pharmaceutical industry in the public sector. Yet, Sokhey was able to broker a USSR offer of technical and financial assistance that enabled India to build pharmaceutical capacity in the public sector. It is interesting to note that the production of pharmaceuticals in India was not under the jurisdiction of the Ministry of Health but within the ambit of the Ministry of Industry. Nehru was attracted to the Soviet model of industrialization as India disembarked on its Five-Year Plans. However, as the Planning Commission was formulating India's Second Five-Year Plan in the mid-fifties, Nehru was concerned because the Plan had envisioned a greater role for the private sector in pharmaceuticals. Although he was not opposed to private-sector participation in the pharmaceutical industry, Nehru was apprehensive with respect to Indian drug companies entering into collaboration with transnational corporations. The transnational corporations insisted that the price of drugs manufactured in collaboration with the local companies should be identical to that of the imported article.[95]

The USSR's offer of technical assistance to India included support for a pharmaceutical complex that included facilities for production of antibiotics such as streptomycin, used in the treatment of TB; vitamins and anti-malarial drugs; and intermediates for drug manufacture. Concerned that commercial interests would stall India's progress in building pharmaceutical self-sufficiency, the Indian ambassador to the USSR sought to gain the support of Nehru for the Soviet venture.[96] But Nehru was wary of continued technological dependence on the USSR and consulted with T.T. Krishnamachari. The latter emphasized that the Soviet scheme be tailored to existing production capacities and the government enable pharmaceutical companies in the private sector to expand in areas where they already had a presence.[97] M.O. Mathai, Nehru's special assistant, suggested that if transnational corporations could provide essential drugs at affordable prices, India could minimize technological dependence on the Soviets.[98]

By September 1957, the Economic Affairs Committee of the Nehru cabinet endorsed the recommendations of the Ministry of Commerce that transnational corporations hold minority shares in Indian pharmaceutical ventures. The Economic Affairs Committee endorsed the Ministry's proposal to seek West German collaboration for the manufacture of dyes, US collaboration for vitamins and synthetic hormones, and Soviet assistance for the manufacture of synthetic drugs.[99] Whereas the Soviets proposed to set up an integrated pharmaceutical plant, the Indian Ministry of Commerce sought an isolated intermediates plant for the production of dyes and pharmaceuticals.

Apart from misgivings about Soviet aid for the Indian pharmaceutical industry, Nehru was equally concerned about the monopoly of Western transnational corporations. In the 1958 edition of *Chemical and Engineering News* of the American Chemical Society, a news article featured the then Finance Minister Morarji Desai's visit to the US. The article noted that since 1956, the Russians began a big push to wean India from dependence on Western pharmaceuticals. Soviet engineers, loans, and technical knowhow were provided to build state-owned industry. The Soviet assistance to the Indian pharmaceutical industry was a potential showcase, portraying communism as the friend of the sick and the disabled.[100] Fortunately, for the Free World, the report continued, Western pharmaceutical firms were not idle. Merck agreed to help the Indian government's Hindustan

Antibiotics build the most modern streptomycin plant in the world.[101] The report concluded that the original Soviet offer of technological assistance to the pharmaceutical sector in India was shelved and the Indian pharmaceutical industry was saved from being a government monopoly.

By 1958, the Cabinet approved the proposal to initiate the production of antibiotics, synthetic drugs, and endocrines with Soviet assistance, which led to the establishment of the Indian Drugs and Pharmaceuticals Limited (IDPL). While IDPL experienced a painful evolution, largely caused by the need for experimentation to negotiate around India's existing patent regime, it grew by the early 1970s into not only a major supplier of antibiotics but also the major support for the private sector pharmaceutical companies that were so critical in providing low-cost drugs to the Indian people.[102]

India's struggle to achieve pharmaceutical self-sufficiency during the 1950s was illustrative of the lack of consensus within Nehru's cabinet. This was particularly evident in T.T. Krishnamachari and Morarji Desai's ideological orientation that was at best, skeptical of USSR's technological advancements. Underlining India's quest for pharmaceutical self-sufficiency were two unanswered questions related to the role of the state: (a) whether drugs would be sold at prices that bore a resemblance to income levels; or (b) whether the price of drugs would be regulated by the market. Whereas Nehru was initially hesitant to accept the Soviet offer of technological assistance for India's pharmaceutical sector, he was equally skeptical about the monopoly of Western transnational corporations. In Nehru's view, a pharmaceutical sector under the leadership of the public sector would disincentivize transnational corporations' monopolization of the industry.

Conclusion

Health in newly decolonized countries including India was influenced by international influences such as the Cold War and domestic factors such as addressing the acute shortage of medical personnel and the attainment of pharmaceutical self-sufficiency. Both led to their own inconsistencies and contradictions. In this chapter, I have examined the dilemma of newly independent India walking a tightrope between its strategic positioning in the Cold War as a non-aligned nation and the domestic quest for self-sufficiency.

Through the prosopographies of Amrit Kaur and Sokhey, I critically examine the appropriation and transformation of international aid in India within the broader Cold War dynamics of the 1950s. At the time, the USSR and its Eastern European allies had withdrawn from the WHO citing ideological differences with the US related to the niche of the state in the provision of health services. Soviet aid to India in public health was non-existent until the early fifties. At the same time, technical assistance to newly decolonized countries such as India and Indonesia in the field of medicine formed the cornerstone of the American Point Four Program that was intended to buttress Asia against the rising tide of communism. On the contrary,

Amrit Kaur sought to use US technical assistance to redress the budgetary shortfall for public health.

Indo-Soviet relations strengthened in 1953 following the death of Stalin, Khruschev's policy of de-Stalinization, and India's leadership of the Asian-African Conference at Bandung. The proverbial Bandung Spirit emphasized technological self-sufficiency of newly decolonized nations and opposition to all forms of colonialism.[103] In the aftermath of Bandung, Soviet involvement with the health sector in India was only incidental and was concerned with the proposal of establishing a drug industry under state auspices. The weakest aspect of Bandung and the non-aligned program was economic development. Although India was successful in building state capacity in the production of pharmaceuticals with Soviet aid and transnational technological collaboration, the West was the source of technological knowhow.[104] The Soviets were unsuccessful in terms of providing an economic alternative to Western capitalist economy except in the defense sector. Very little of the economic development agenda put forward by India and other non-aligned nations at the Asian-African Conference at Bandung, particularly economic self-sufficiency, was ever agreed upon multilaterally or implemented in practice. Domestic factors in other countries—particularly the end of the Soekarno Era in Indonesia (1965), following the September 30 Movement that resulted in the country being drawn into Western orbit—militated against the Bandung Spirit. On the domestic front, although India was successful in reducing the prices of drugs, similar success was not evident in the case of transforming medical education.

Acknowledgments

Thanks are due to Corinna R. Unger, David Engerman, Robert Smith, Mangesh Kulkarni, Vivek Neelakantan, Dr. Mohan B Dikshit, Radhika Hegde, and Mallika Kavadi for sharing or procuring reprints, photocopies of articles and photographs. The article draws upon two projects for which research and travel grants were received from the Rockefeller Archive Centre, Sir Dorabji Tata Trust, and the Wellcome Trust. Most importantly my gratitude to Vivek for his consideration, patience, encouragement, incisive criticisms, and substantial editing of the manuscript when the writing got tough with several health issues that plagued me.

Notes

1 See Radhika Ramasubban, *Public Health and Medical Research in India: Their Origins Under the Impact of British Colonial Policy* (Stockholm: Swedish Agency for Research Cooperation, Sarec Report, 1982); David Arnold, *Colonizing the Body, State Medicine and Epidemic Disease in Nineteenth Century India* (Delhi: Oxford University Press, 1993); Mark Harrison, *Public Health in British India: Anglo Indian Preventive Medicine 1859–1914* (New Delhi: Foundation Books, 1994); Mridula Ramanna, *Western Medicine and Public Health in Colonial Bombay 1845–1895* (New Delhi: Orient Longman, 2002).

2 Shirish N. Kavadi, *Rockefeller Foundation and Public Health in Colonial India, 1916–1945: A Narrative History* (Mumbai/Pune: The Foundation for Research in Community Health, 1999); See also Shirish N. Kavadi, "Rockefeller Public Health in Colonial India," in *Histories of Medicine and Healing in the Indian Ocean World,* vol. 2, Anna Winterbottom and Facil Tesfaye edited (Basingstoke: Palgrave Macmillan, 2016), 61–88.

3 Shirish N. Kavadi, "Medicine, Philanthropy and Nationhood: Tensions of Different Visions in India," in *Public Health and National Reconstruction in Post-War Asia: International Influences, Local Transformations,* Liping Bu and Ka-Che Yip edited (Abingdon, Oxon: Routledge, 2014), 132–153.

4 Nasir Tyabji, "Negotiating Nonalignment Dilemmas Attendant on Initiating Pharmaceutical Production in India," *Technology and Culture* 53 (2012): 37–60; see also Nasir Tyabji, "Gaining Technical Know-How in an Unequal World: Penicillin Manufacture in Nehru's India," *MPRA Paper No 84236* (2004), https://mpra.ub.uni-muenchen.de/84236; Nasir Tyabji, "Aligning with Both the Soviet Union and with the Pharmaceutical Transnationals: Dilemmas Attendant on Initiating Drug Production in India, *ISID Working Paper* 2010/08 (New Delhi: ISID, 2010), 1–26.

5 David Arnold, "Colonial Medicine in Transition: Medical Research in India, 1910–14," *South Asia Research* 14 (1994): 10–35; Pratik Chakrabarti "Signs of the Times": Medicine and Nationhood in British India," *Osiris* 24 (2009): 188–211; Sunil Amrith, "Political Culture of Health in India: A Historical Perspective," *Economic and Political Weekly* XLII (2007): 114–121.

6 Ashish Bose, "Health Policy in India," in *Policy Making in India*, Madan K. D. edited (New Delhi: GoI, 1982); Roger Jeffery, *The Politics of Health in India* (Berkeley: University of California Press, 1988), 246.

7 Kalikinkar Sengupta, "The Bhore Committee Report and Thereafter," *Science and Culture* 13 (1947): 187.

8 Editorial, "Medical Education in India," *Calcutta Medical Journal* (1948): 440–441. See also Kavadi, "Medicine, Philanthropy and Nationhood.

9 David Arnold, "Nehruvian Science and Postcolonial India," *ISIS* 104 (2013): 370–380; See also Nasir Tyabji, "Jawaharlal Nehru and Science and Technology," *Contemporary Perspectives* 1, no. 1 (January to June 2007): 130–136.

10 Kris Manjapra, "Knowledgeable Internationalism and the Swadeshi Movement, 1930–1921," *Economic and Political Weekly* XLVII (2012): 53.

11 Arnold, "Nehruvian Science," 366.

12 Prabir Purukayastha, The Untold Story of the Left in Indian Science, *Peoples Democracy* (2020), https://peoplesdemocracy.in/2020/1018_pd/untold-story-left-indian-science.

13 "Harkishan Singh, "Sahib Singh Sokhey (1887–1971): An Eminent Medico-Pharmaceutical Professional," *Indian Journal of History of Science* 51, no. 2 (2016): 238–247.

14 Purukayastha, "The Untold Story of the Left in Indian Science."

15 Ibid.

16 Nikhil Menon, *Planning Democracy. How a Professor, An Institute and an Idea Shaped India* (Gurugram: Penguin Random House India, 2022), x.

17 See Robert S. Anderson, *Nucleus and Nation: Scientists, International Networks, and Power in India* (New Delhi: Supernova Publishers, 2011).

18 See for example Vivek Neelakantan, "The Campaign Against the Big Four Endemic Diseases and Indonesia's Engagement with the Cold War 1950s," in *Public Health and National Reconstruction in Post-War Asia: International Influences, Local Transformations*, Liping Bu and Ka-Che Yip edited (Abingdon: Routledge, 2014), 154–174.

19 David C. Engerman, *The Price of Aid: The Economic Cold War in India* (Cambridge, MA: Harvard University Press, 2018).

20 Manu Bhagawan, "Introduction," in *India and the Cold War*, Manu Bhagawan edited (Gurugram: Penguin Random House India, 2019), 10.

21 David C. Engerman, "South Asia and the Cold War," in *The Cold War in the Third World*, Robert McMohon edited (Oxford: Oxford University Press, 2013) 67–83.

22 Sushila Nayyar, "Rajkumari Amrit Kaur," *Rajkumari Amrit Kaur: Eminent Parliamentarians Monograph Series* 15 (New Delhi: Lok Sabha Secretariat, 1993), 27–33.

23 Ibid., 31.

24 Emily Rook-Koepsel, "Constructing Women's Citizenship: The Local, National, and Global Civics Lessons of Rajkumari Amrit Kaur," *Journal of Women's History* 27 (2015): 154–175.

25 C. G. Pandit, *My World of Preventive Medicine* (New Delhi: Indian Council of Medical Research, 1995); R. L. Bijlani, "All India Institute of Medical Sciences New Delhi," *The National Medical Journal of India* 6 (1999): 181–186; Shirish N. Kavadi, "Autonomy for Medical Institutes in India: A View From History," *The National Medical Journal of India* 30 (2017): 230–234; V. Srinivas, "Raj Kumari Amrit Kaur," *AIIMS Diamond Jubilee Celebrations* (New Delhi: AIIMS, 2016).

26 Bijlani All India Institute of Medical Sciences, 1999; Srinivas Raj Kumari Amrit Kaur, 2016.

27 Kavadi, "Medicine, Philanthropy and Nationhood."

28 See for example Jeffery, *The Politics of Health in India.*

29 See for example Marshall C. Balfour, "Diary Notes," May 1954, Officers' Diaries, RG 12, Rockefeller Archive Center (RAC).

30 Kaur to Dean Rusk, July 31, 1956, Projects RG 1.2, Series 460, Box 1, Folder 2, RAC.

31 Kavadi, "Medicine, "Philanthropy and Nationhood."

32 Elizabeth Fee, Theodore Brown and Marcos Cueto, "At the Roots of The World Health Organization's Challenges: Politics and Regionalization," *American Journal of Public Health* 106, no. 11 (2016): 1912–1917.

33 John A. Logan, "Counteracting Communism Through Foreign Assistance Programs in Public Health," *American Journal of Public Health* 45 (1955): 1017–1021; see also Chester Bowles, *Ambassador's Report* (New York: Harper and Brothers, 1954).

34 Manjapra, "Knowledgeable Internationalism."

35 Leonard A. Gordon, "Wealth Equals Wisdom? The Rockefeller and Ford Foundations in India," *Annals of the American Academy of Political and Social Science* 554 (1997): 104.

36 Jeffery, *The Politics of Health in India.*

37 Ibid.

38 Ibid.

39 Ibid.

40 Ibid.

41 Ibid.

42 Ibid.

43 Ibid.

44 Ibid.

45 Ibid.

46 "The Health Ministry's Budget for 1949–50," *Calcutta Medical Journal* (November 1949): 359.

47 Ibid.

48   Kavadi, "Medicine, Philanthropy and Nationhood."
49   C. G. Pandit, and K. Someswara Rao, *Indian Research Fund Association and Indian Council of Medical Research, 1911–1961: Fifty Years of Progress* (New Delhi: Indian Council of Medical Research, 1961), 206.
50   "Presidential Address at the All-India Medical Conference, Trivandrum: Dr C.S. Thakar," *Calcutta Medical Journal* (1957): n.p.
51   "Nehru to Krishnamachari," August 26, 1957, *Selected Works of Jawaharlal Nehru: August 1–October 31, 1957*, vol. 39, Mushirul Hasan edited (New Delhi: Jawaharlal Nehru Memorial Fund, 2007), 21.
52   Jeffery, *The Politics of Health in India*; Kavadi, "Medicine, Philanthropy and Nationhood"; Amrith, "Political Culture of Health in India"; Rushikesh M. Maru, "Policy Formulation as Political Process: A Case Study of Health Manpower: 1949–75," in *Public Policy and Policy Analysis in India*, R. S. Ganapathy et al. edited (New Delhi: Sage Publications, 1985), 150–177.
53   Maru, "Policy Formulation as Political Process."
54   John Farley, *To Cast Out Disease: A History of the International Health Division of the Rockefeller Foundation, 1913–1951* (New York: Oxford University Press, 2004), 278.
55   Grant to M. C. Balfour, November 20, 1944, General Correspondence, RG2, Series 464, Box 275, F 1884, RAC.
56   "Comments on Methods of Selection of the Fellows in Medicine and Public Health in India," New Delhi Field Office, RG 6.7, Series 1, Box 138, F 990; "Anderson to Rusk," July 31, 1958, Projects, RG 1.2, S 460, Box 1, F 2, RAC.
57   "Grant to M.C. Balfour," November 20, 1944, General Correspondence, RG 2, Series 464, Box 275, F 1884, RAC.
58   Undated, "Notes on Discussion: India Conference," RAC.
59   For a comparison with Indonesia see also Vivek Neelakantan, "The Expansion and Transformation of Medical Education in Indonesia During the 1950s in Jakarta and Surabaya," in *Translating the Body: Medical Education in Southeast Asia*, in Hans Pols, C. Michele Thompson and John Harley Warner edited (Singapore: NUS Press, 2017), 173–193. Neelakantan contends that during the 1950s, Indonesia refashioning its medical curricula based on the curricula extant in North American schools was a part of the geopolitical strategy of the US and philanthropic foundations such as the Rockefeller Foundation and the China Medical Board to win the loyalty of the Indonesian leadership in the fight against communism.
60   "Note to Secretary General, Exchange schemes between India and USA," April 14, 1954, *Selected Works of Jawaharlal Nehru: February 1, 1954–May 31, 1954* vol. 25, Ravinder Kumar and Sharada Prasad edited (New Delhi: Jawaharlal Nehru Memorial Fund, 1999).
61   Manjapra, "Knowledgeable Internationalism and the Swadeshi Movement," 53.
62   Jeffery, *The Politics of Health in India*, 246.
63   "Correspondence between Nehru to Morarji Desai," May 13, 1953, *Selected Works of Jawaharlal Nehru: April 1, 1953–June 30, 1953* vol. 22, Ravinder Kumar and Sharada Prasad edited (New Delhi: Nehru Memorial Fund, 1998), 366.
64   Nehru to Deshmukh May 7, 1953; Note to Secretary General, Ministry of External Affairs, May 6, 1953; "To Cabinet Secretary, Engagement of Foreign Experts, May 9, 1953, *Selected Works of Jawaharlal Nehru, April 1–June 30, 1953* vol. 22, Ravinder Kumar and Sharada Prasad edited (New Delhi: Jawaharlal Nehru Memorial Fund, 1998), 131–132, 353, 300.
65   "Friedgood to Gregg," August 23, 1953, *Alan Gregg Papers*, MSC 190, Box 16, National Library of Medicine, Bethesda.

66 "Secretary, Ministry of Education, GoI to the Vice Chancellor, Lucknow University," December 21, 1956, Projects, RG 1.2, S 460, Box 1, F 2, RAC.
67 "Kaur to Rusk," July 31, 1956, Projects, RG 1.2, S 460, Box 1, F 2, RAC.
68 Ibid.
69 "Alan Gregg to Kaur," June 13, 1953, Projects, RG 1.2, S 464, Box 44, F 386, RAC.
70 "Kaur to Gregg," June 18, 1953, Projects, RG 1.2, S 464, Box 44, F 386, RAC.
71 The Colombo Plan had its origins in a conference held in Colombo, Ceylon in 1950. In Southeast Asia, the British in the aftermath of World War II sought to reconcile local nationalism with external interests. The British were apprehensive that as old-fashioned nationalism in Southeast Asia would give way to communism, the region needed to be buttressed against the tide of communism. To this end, the Colombo Plan introduced a program of technical assistance for Southeast Asia. For details refer Nicholas Tarling, "The United Kingdom and the Origins of the Colombo Plan," *The Journal of Commonwealth and Comparative Politics* 24, no. 1 (2008): 3–34.
72 Shirish N. Kavadi, "Autonomy for Medical Institutes in India: A View from History," *National Medical Journal of India* 30 (2017): 230–234.
73 Jeffery, *The Politics of Health in India.*
74 Ibid.
75 Ibid.
76 Kavadi, "Medicine, Philanthropy and Nationhood," 2015.
77 Vijay Singh, "Some Strategies of Indian Communists after 1947, in *India in the World since 1947: National and Transnational Perspectives,* Andreas Hilger and Corinna R. Unger edited (Frankfurt: Peter Lang, 2012), 99–119; Swapna Kona Nayudu, "The Soviet Peace Offensive and Nehru's India, 1953–1956," in *India and the Cold War,* Manu Bhagawan edited (Gurugram: Penguin Random House India, 2019).
78 Nayudu, "The Soviet Peace Offensive and Nehru's India."
79 Ibid.
80 For details see A. Lakshmana Chetty, "India and the 1954 Geneva Conference," *Proceedings of the Indian History Congress* 39, no. 2 (1978): 618–626.
81 Bhagawan, *India and the Cold War.*
82 Ibid.
83 Andreas Hilger, "Building a Socialist Elite?: Khrushchev's Soviet Union and Elite Formation in India," *in Elites and Decolonization in the Twentieth Century,* Jost Dulffer and Marc Frey edited (Basingstoke: Palgrave MacMillan, 2011), 262–286.
84 Ibid.
85 See also Jan Carew, *Green Winter. A Novel About a Negro Student in Moscow Today* (New York: Berkeley Medallion Books, 1966).
86 Purukayastha, The Untold Story of the Left in Indian Science, 2020.
87 Ibid.
88 Singh, "Sahib Singh Sokhey (1887–1971)."
89 Ibid.
90 Dominique A. Tobbell, "Who's Winning the Human Race?" Cold War as Pharmaceutical Political Strategy, *Journal of the History of Medicine and Allied Sciences* 64 (2009): 429–473.
91 Ibid.
92 Tyabji, "Negotiating Nonalignment Dilemmas," 42.
93 Ibid., 38.
94 Ibid., 40.

95   See also "Letter from Nehru to T. T. Krishnamachari, "October 8, 1955, in *Selected Works of Jawaharlal Nehru: September 1–November 30 1955*, vol. 30, H. Y. Sharada Prasad and A. K. Damodaran edited (New Delhi: Jawaharlal Nehru Memorial Fund, 2002), 196.

96   Tyabji, "Negotiating Nonalignment Dilemmas," 41.

97   Ibid., 42.

98   Ibid., 52.

99   Ibid., 53.

100 "Merck Moves into India: Merck's Entry in Indian Pharmaceuticals Makes Friends, Future Profits, and Helps Sideswipe Soviets," *Chemical & Engineering News* 36 (November 1958): 73.

101 Ibid.

102 Tyabji, "Aligning with both the Soviet Union and with the Pharmaceutical Transnationals", https://mpra.ub.uni-muenchen.de/79240/.

103 For the Indonesian context, see for example Vivek Neelakantan, *Science, Public Health and Nation-Building in Soekarno-Era Indonesia* (Newcastle-upon-Tyne: Cambridge Scholars Publishing, 2017).

104 See also Shivshankar Menon, *India and Asian Geopolitics: The Past, Present* (New York: Brookings Institution Press, 2021).

3 Malaria Eradication and Modernization in the Maldives and Sri Lanka, 1941–84

Eva-Maria Knoll

Introduction

The fight against malaria in the Maldives provides a remarkable exception regarding temporality and outcome in a prominent international health activity of the twentieth century. This effort transformed Malaria, the tropical disease par excellence[1] "from an imperial disease that tested governance over 'tropical' peoples into an issue of international health politics and nation-state building."[2] Entangled in Cold War ideologies and emancipation aspirations of the colonized, the WHO's unilateral vertical disease elimination strategy had been shifting in the 1960s to a rather horizontal strategy of "multisectoral policies that integrated anti-malaria programmes in national health services."[3]

The historian Randall Packard has elaborated on the politically strategic and technology-driven bias and shortcomings of these campaigns. Especially the malaria eradication program lacked "flexibility and adaptability, developed poor planning without knowing the social, cultural and administrative challenges that it faced."[4] Yet the small island communities of the Maldives succeeded while this international health effort had failed in many other parts of the globe. In 2015 the WHO formally certified the Maldives as the first malaria-free country in the WHO South-East Asia Region (SEARO). What thereby became conspicuous in fact represents a staggering sustained achievement, since the archipelago looks back at a pronounced feverish history. Written records document 600 years of the deadly impact of "Maldive fevers." Nevertheless, this archipelago came comparatively late into the focus of the global malaria eradication program launched in the post-WWII period.

Located at the crossroads of Indian Ocean trade and shipping routes in monsoon Asia and in proximity to the complex disease environments of India and Sri Lanka (the historical Ceylon), the Maldives had always been entangled in the Indian Ocean World's "disease zone."[5] Yet the archipelago has a distinct health trajectory shaped by trans-local entanglements in colonial and post-colonial geopolitics, by its distinct environment of 1192 low-lying coral islands, and by the settlement structure of this littoral

DOI: 10.4324/9781003332060-4

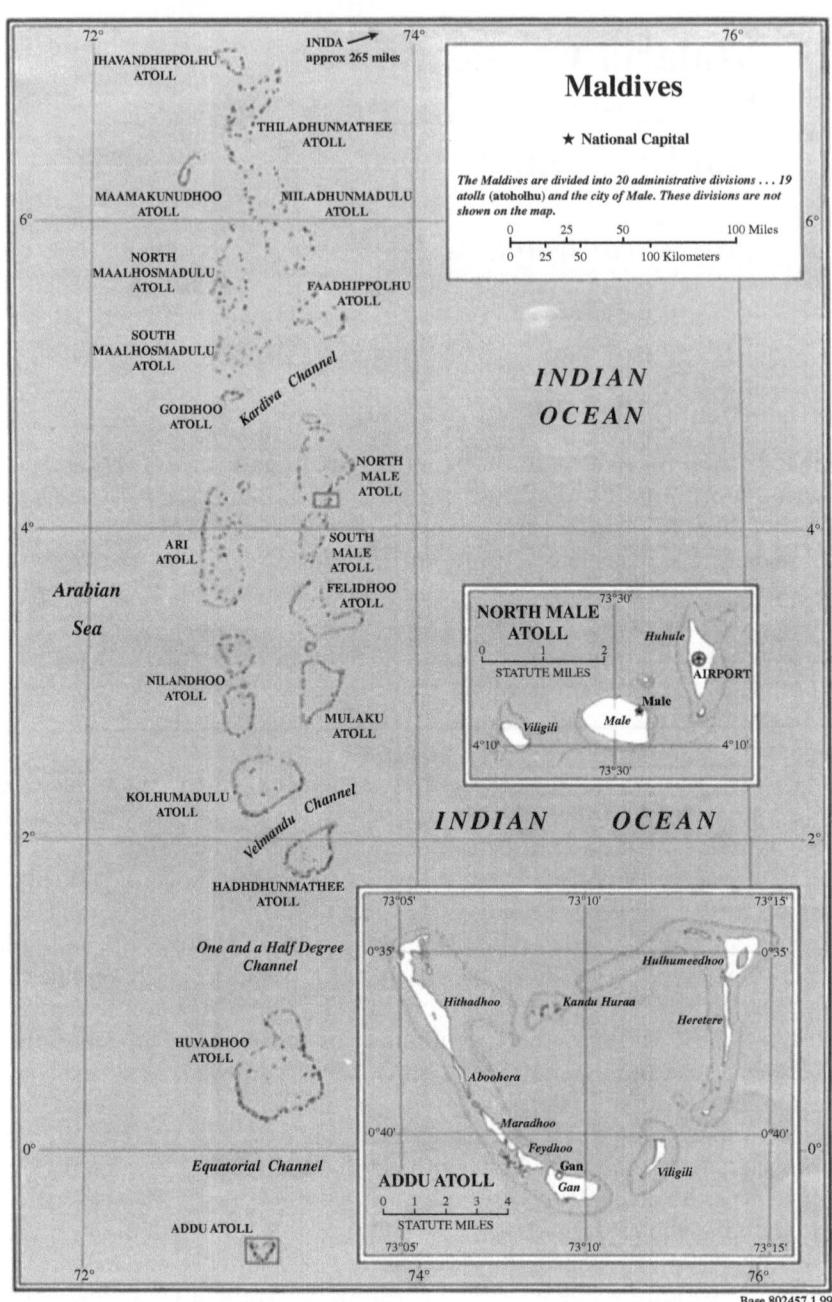

Map 3.1 Map of the Maldives (1998)

Credit: US Central Intelligence Agency (1998)
The image is in the public domain:
https://commons.wikimedia.org/wiki/File:Maldives_pol98.jpg.

society, living—until the advent of tourism—from subsistence fishing and cross-oceanic trade dispersed in small population pockets across about 200 islands.

Tracing the successful fight of a small and remote island nation, often overlooked in South Asian scholarship, against one of humanity's deadliest diseases, this chapter investigates: a) why a global public health effort arrived comparatively late in the center of the Indian Ocean; and b) why this belated eradication effort was exceptionally successful in the Maldives. It thereby highlights local viewpoints and some of the geopolitical entanglements of this disease eradication trajectory and the more general health developments in the island nation.

When SEARO was established in 1948 as WHO's first regional office, the Maldives archipelago still was a sultanate under British protection. In 1953, the UK represented the Maldive islands as an Associate Member in the SEARO until 1965, when the islands became independent.[6] During the 1950s, the SEARO developed short-term demonstration projects—with particular reference to the control of malaria, TB, and venereal diseases—as training grounds where the SEARO staff would work with local personnel and help them learn new techniques to solve health problems. Prior to independence (1965), filariasis was a major public health concern in the Maldives. In 1951, on behalf of the Maldive islands, the UK government requested technical assistance in the eradication of the disease. The WHO appointed Dr. M.O.T. Iyengar as a short-term Filariasis Consultant. Iyengar noted that endemic filariasis and malaria were rampant in the Maldive islands at the time.[7] Malnutrition was common. In the Suvadiva and Addu atolls, for example, the recorded death rates were higher than the birth rates.[8] The WHO team led by Iyengar carried out epidemiological surveys of filariasis and malaria. The findings revealed a general dearth of public health facilities, except on the island of Malé.

In 1966, post-war approaches to modernization also reached the remote Maldive islands, and finally, a malaria-eradication program was launched there at a time when the WHO's overly ambitious Global Malaria Eradication Program was, in fact, already being withdrawn. Small and insignificant in size of territory, population, and exploitable resources, the island nation often was overlooked and neglected in the geopolitics of South Asia and by scholarly attention. The archipelago thus lagged behind in health developments—although the Maldives were a nominal British crown protectorate with internal self-government from 1887 until 1965—and despite close political and epidemiological interactions with India and Sri Lanka (the historical Ceylon). This chapter investigates in what ways and why the Maldive islands were remarkable in the global history of malaria eradication. For this purpose, the local late-colonial history and postcolonial history of malaria eradication efforts in the Maldives will be contrasted against the different cases in Sri Lanka. Unlike partially successful, failed, and rebounding efforts in neighboring India and Sri Lanka as well as in many other parts of the malaria-ridden world, the eradication of vectors and parasites succeeded in the Maldives.

The present analysis reveals the kind of successful adaptation of the general WHO eradication strategy to local circumstances that had been criticized as missing for other parts of the world. The small-scale geographical and biosocial circumstances of the Maldivian archipelago—notably, a small and dispersed population in an infrastructure-weak setting—presented the eradication program with enormous challenges. Yet small island settings had proven advantageous in terms of quarantine and isolation in the history of fighting infectious diseases, and the interplay of global and regional with national and local structures, factors, and agencies worked out in this case. Moreover, in times of a collapsing colonial Indian Ocean world, the dawn of independence for India and Sri Lanka enhanced the geopolitical strategic location of the Maldives as a stopover midway between the Middle East and the Far East. Though the Maldives gained independence from the United Kingdom on July 26, 1965, a Royal Air Force base was in use in the southernmost atoll until 1975. The small hospital of the RAF base on Gan Island provided early biomedical services in the region. The RAF airfield closed when the geopolitical interests of the UK and the US shifted to Diego Garcia and the Chagos archipelago some 750 km further south. The ongoing dispute over the maritime borders and the respective exclusive economic zones (EEZ) between the two neighboring archipelagos, however, still entangles the Maldives to an extent in the long breath of continuing decolonization struggles between the Chagossian islanders, Mauritius, and the UK. At the same time, the archipelago is intertwined with the intensifying geopolitical and postcolonial rivalry between India and China in the Indian Ocean. It has gained worldwide significance on an unprecedented scale as the central maritime highway for the global economy. This article discusses the post-war and post-colonial health history of the Maldives within changing contexts—located in the center of the Indian Ocean and on the fringe of the WHO South East-Asia Region—that have remained central to global health developments since its foundation.

A Case Temporally Inconsistent with the Historiography of Malaria Eradication

In 1955, at the Eighth World Health Assembly in Mexico City, the WHO decided on an aggressive intervention counting on dichlorodiphenyltrichloroethane (DDT), later known as the "vertical approach." Its goal was to interrupt transmission for 3–5 years in order to eliminate malaria before mosquitoes developed resistance to the chemical.[9] The "complex web of technical expertise, humanitarian motivations, economic interests, and political will" that was spun to initiate and fuel malaria eradication as "the largest international health program of the second half of the twentieth century"[10] was subjected to critical analysis. Scholars scrutinized the origins, rise, and decline of vertical disease eradication efforts, notably their anchoring in colonial structures and Cold War ideologies, their entanglements in development, modernization, decolonization, and public health discourses, and the implications for developing countries and postcolonial states.[11]

In the 1960s, it had become clear that malaria eradication could not be achieved in the near future—though it remained as the ultimate goal.[12] In 1969, the global malaria eradication campaign was formally ended. Ever since, programs to control and to eradicate malaria have coexisted.[13] Strategies in international medicine shifted from targeting specific diseases for elimination with universal "magic bullets" toward primary healthcare to address the diseases' socio-economic complexity.[14] The post-World War II era thus allows for the identification of two competing approaches to disease eradication. Both approaches were characterized by Cold War rivalry, notably by concerns that newly independent nations in developing Asia might fall to communism. Cold War ideology shaped international aid and development strategies in a sequential manner. By the second half of the 1960s, the narrow, vertical biomedical approach of the earlier phase, counting on technological solutions such as DDT, mass medication, and vaccination, had shifted toward a holistic horizontal approach concerned with raising general living and health standards.[15] In the scholarly study of man's struggle against malaria, health historian Kalinga Tudor Silva identified three different approaches. One, the "modernist approach," based on a scientific understanding of the disease. Two, the "history of colonial medicine" that infuses a colonial objective by featuring natives as the infectious and resistant "other" in malaria control. Three, a "socio-historical perspective" that includes traditional knowledge systems.[16]

Against these backgrounds and with their distinctive febrile history, the Maldives can be seen as a showcase in the global malaria eradication campaign and in its scholarly reflections. The economic development of tourism and fisheries following the progressive reduction of cases corroborates the malaria-blocks-development thesis.[17] The successful and lasting eradication of malarial vectors and parasites proves the WHO's aggressive vertical approach to be right and feasible. Yet, precisely in view of these accomplishments, the Maldivian showcase does not seem to fit into the global historiography of malaria eradication. By this exceptional status, the course taken by the Maldives apparently differed from the general currents of the international eradication program and its regional application. Despite six hundred documented years of Maldive fever, the Maldives were left behind in the malaria eradication strategy that the WHO SEARO had launched in the region between 1957 and 1961.[18]

600 Documented Years of Maldive Fever

The earliest eye-witness report in the Maldives' centuries-spanning fever history is provided by Ibn Battuta (1304–68/1369), who served as the royal judge in Malé and barely survived the fever attacks.[19] François Pyrard de

Laval (1578–1621), a chronicler in a French merchant expedition to the East Indies and shipwrecked in the islands in 1602, was convinced that every foreign visitor inevitably must catch this "severe and very troublesome" malady "known through all the Indies under the name of Maldive fever."[20] Negotiating for weeks over the purchase of cowry shells in 1723, the crew of a Dutch ship was "one after the other felled by fever," including both commanders.[21] In 1922, the Archaeological Commissioner of Ceylon, H.C.P. Bell (1851–1937), reported from this third visit to the Maldives "no less than three hundred (300) victims, Noble and plebian [sic!] alike, perished from this scourge,"[22] which was about five percent of the capital's population of 6127 (census from 1921).[23] Increased body temperature can have many causes in equatorial latitudes, including vector-transmitted parasites. Nevertheless, most scholars assume the malady described across six centuries as severe "Maldive fever" was virulent malaria.[24]

Mr. Ismail (a pseudonym), one of my local interlocutors, remembers fevers, coughing, and runny noses as the most common types of illness of his childhood. Born in 1945, he grew up in the Maldives' capital island Malé and became a high-ranking civil servant. When he was a boy, high fever was commonly treated by administering water sanctified with recitations from the Quran. As fever was also linked to superstitious beliefs, many would opt for *fanditha* (magical practices) and *thaveedh* (amulets) to keep them safe. Mr. Ismail was still a boy when fevers were attributed to ordinary tiny insects and the notion of malaria became widely known with the arrival of a WHO consultant in the capital island Malé in 1963. Yet at that time, he emphasizes, the southernmost atoll of Addu had already been fogged by chemicals to repel mosquitoes. Like many others, Mr. Ismail remembers the introduction of biomedicine and malaria control in the Maldives correctly as being intertwined with colonial and post-colonial geopolitics.[25] Only when the Maldives were transferred on the global geopolitical map from the neglected fringe of the British Empire toward its center by being turned into a hub for World War II logistics, were bugs targeted as potential disease-transmitting agents. Thus the island sultanate became connected to the international health landscape.

A Belated Start: Malaria Eradication
in a Remote Island Nation

Malaria is a life-threatening disease caused by a single-cell protozoan parasite (*Plasmodium*) and transmitted in a complex two-stage cycle in humans and species of *Anopheles* mosquitoes. An infected female *Anopheles* transmits the parasite through saliva when stinging.[26] Malaria surveys from the second half of the twentieth century shed new light on the 600 years of documented raging fevers that haunted a remote island people with a largely independent history.

The islands had been settled for about 2,500 years, linking the origins of the *Dhivehin* (as Maldivians call themselves) to the Indian subcontinent and Sri Lanka. Throughout most of its history the Dhivehin had been an independent but well-connected island people in their mid-oceanic location. Their involvement in Islamic networks intensified when the Maldives officially embraced the Muslim faith in 1153 CE. A brief period of Portuguese dominance from 1558 to 1573, recorded in local memory as extremely brutal, was the early historical exception in direct colonial rule. The victory over the Portuguese in a guerrilla war is commemorated as the Maldives National Day. Throughout the remaining colonial period, however, the Maldives were nominally a protectorate, though largely retaining self-government in accordance with Islamic rules and paying annual tributes for protection in matters of foreign policy: to the Dutch from 1645, to the French in the mid-eighteenth century, and to the British via Ceylon from 1796.[27] Certified in 1887, this nominal though rather loose connection to the British Empire ended officially in 1965 when the Maldives gained independence. The extractive colonial British regime was focusing on fertile and prospering Ceylon and India and left the small, sandy, sparsely populated, fever-ridden Maldive islands, which were above all difficult to navigate, largely to themselves—also in health matters. The Maldives with their proud history of independence, in turn, were conveniently remote to colonial sovereignty and thus also somewhat reluctant to accept colonial and international health interventions.

Early entomological research recorded 15 mosquito species in five atolls, two of them of the genus *Anopheles*, and multiple breeding grounds, including lakes, mangroves, taro fields, tanks, and wells.[28] The equatorial location comes with meteorological conditions that are "optimum for the activities of the anopheles vectors and consequent transmission of malaria throughout the year."[29] It became clear that the Maldive islands were a mixed infection zone where humans were vulnerable to three malaria parasites: *Plasmodium falciparum* and *Plasmodium vivax* (which accounted for about half of all infections) and *Plasmodium malariae*.[30] Especially those with a naive immune system were hit hard, notably children and visiting foreigners. A WHO "reflection of the intensity of transmission (...) prior to commencement of control measures (...) was that nearly 50 percent of the children had malaria parasites in their blood."[31] Despite this pronounced risk of infection, the archipelago came comparatively late into the focus of the global malaria eradication efforts.

A Crumbling Empire Meets Small Malicious Bugs: An Early Phase of Repelling Febrile Disease in the Maldives

The history of repelling febrile disease and its causative vectors in the Maldive islands displays two distinctive phases. The first phase was entangled in war logistics. It had its focus in the southernmost fringe of the archipelago and not, as one might aspect, in the capital of Malé, the historic Sultan's island, located as the political and socio-economic heart of the island nation in the very center of the archipelago stretching over 870 km. In fall 1941, a battalion of 1059 Royal Marines was badly affected by the endemic scrub typhus fever while clearing Gan Island in Addu Atoll of any vegetation in order to construct an airfield on this southernmost tip of the archipelago.[32] The dawning independence of India and Ceylon left the disintegrating British Empire in Asia in need of a replacement for its staging posts enroute to the Far East. More than 11,000 palm trees were cleared and Gan's local population was resettled to neighboring islands. The British troops recorded 42 scrub typhus cases from October to December 1941, followed by 582, 382, and 92 cases in the next 3 years.[33] During WWII "scrub typhus emerged out to be the most dreaded disease among the soldiers of the Far East."[34] It "was the most notable rickettsiosis affecting US troops and had a higher mortality rate than any other infectious disease in WWII in the China-Burma-India theatre of operations."[35] Scrub typhus, a febrile disease with mild to life-threatening manifestations, is caused by the *Orientia tsutsugamushi* (formerly *Rickettsia*) pathogen and transmitted by larval mites or "chiggers" of the Trombiculidae family feeding on blood, usually of small rodents. Scrub typhus is endemic in Asia and the most common re-emerging Rickettsial infection in the SEARO region.[36]

A tented hospital of 20 beds, set up in 1941 in Gan for the Royal Navy, was the Maldives' first biomedical health facility. The devastating outbreak of scrub typhus fever demanded a swift expansion to 90 beds and additional support by H.M. Hospital Ship *Vita* and Hospital Ship *Ophir*. In 1943 this was replaced by a more permanent structure.[37] Even after the years of independence for Sri Lanka, Pakistan, and India, the Maldives' south with Gan as its center of gravity remained the British focus of attention for arthropod diseases. Early surveys were rather carried out to safeguard the British military foothold in the region than to tackle a public health problem in the whole archipelago. These early entomological surveys were carried out by a WHO team in 1951, focusing on malaria and on lymphatic filariasis, commonly known as elephantiasis, another major mosquito-borne disease in the islands.[38]

In 1957, the airfield became the Royal Air Force Station Gan, commonly known as RAF Gan. With the extended runway stretching across its entire length, Gan Island has "from the air the appearance of some huge, green, misshapen aircraft carrier"[39] and with its deep-water lagoon, Gan was also ideal for naval refueling.[40] In the Maldives' health history, RAF Gan thus became a crucial place for constituting "the medical" in a co-production of medicine and socio-political worlds.[41] Some 800–900 Maldivians were employed alongside about 100–200 Pakistanis to work for the 600 RAF personnel in Gan. The RAF workforce and locals from neighboring islands in Addu Atoll were the first Maldivians benefiting from biomedical services offered in the RAF hospital. "We see about 1,100 Maldivians a month" explained Surgeon Flight Lieutenant Martin Ward, "and perform 40 to 50 operations, 80 percent of which are on Maldivians."[42]

Although the Maldives had nominally been a British protectorate since 1887, the Royal Naval Medical Service arrived in 1941 only when the constraints of WWII and of the late colonial period seemed to require it, with sparse health information for the airfield operation. Cases of elephantiasis had been observed among the islanders and malaria was suspected.[43] "The enlarged spleens of chronic malaria" were also observed in the local population[44] and "malaria of all types, but with benign tertian predominating" ranked next to the outbreak of scrub typhus and next to diphtheria, bacillary dysentery, chronic skin ulcerations, and gastroenteritis among the diseases responsible for the high incidence of sickness among the Naval forces.[45] For the early war years the report noted: "antimalarial precautions left much to be desired. (...) The breeding of mosquitoes was little reduced by the spraying of pools in the camp areas, and it was obvious that large scale engineering measures were really necessary to be of real use." An "entomological party from Colombo" directed measures toward *Anopheles tessellatus* mosquitoes and "by September 1943 anophelenes [sic!] were greatly reduced in number with a falling off in the incidence of malaria" [46] in Addu Atoll.

About 7 years after the Royal Navy treated soldiers and locals in hospital tents in Gan Island, during the WHO foundation year of 1948, the first biomedical center called *Hasfathaal* opened in the capital island of Malé.[47] As Mr. Ismail mentioned above, when a WHO consultant arrived in Malé to prepare for a malaria eradication program in 1963, the southernmost atoll of Addu had already been sprayed some 20 years earlier.

Fighting Malaria in Islands Big and Small: Near-Eradication and Setbacks in Sri Lanka

In May 1966, with WHO assistance, the Maldives launched the national Malaria Eradication Program, a year after the island nation obtained independence and about 3 years after near-eradication had already been achieved in neighboring Sri Lanka. In view of their close socio-economic and political entanglements in the twentieth century, this timing discrepancy requires a brief comparison of malaria control in the two South Asian Island states. This may appear courageous because they could hardly be more different. Sri Lanka has 200 times the land area of the Maldives (298 km^2) while being about five times as densely populated. When malaria eradication started in 1966, the Maldives had a resident population of 100,883,[48] Sri Lanka some 11.38 million. Environmental constraints are all too obvious in the small low-lying coral islands of the Maldives, a country that is 99% ocean, with very limited soil for cultivation. By contrast, manmade environmental constrains had the largest impact in the malaria hyperendemic Dry Zone of agrarian Sri Lanka.[49]

Since Ceylon was subject to the rationale of developing a plantation economy, scientific research on malaria began in the early twentieth century. Systematic anti-malaria campaigns had started in this British Crown colony as early as 1911[50] and gained momentum after the 1934/35 epidemic with its estimated 80–100,000 deaths.[51] By 1947 Ceylon had become "the first country in Asia to apply DDT as a residual insecticide spraying houses." Malaria morbidity and mortality showed a marked decline from 1.7 m infections in 1944 to 17 cases by 1963—local transmission was almost eliminated.[52] Yet that phase of near eradication was followed by resurgence, when progress in malaria control became entangled with Sinhala nationalist ideology and political ambition.[53] Meanwhile, chronic poverty persisted and development did not ease but aggravated the malaria problem.[54] Residual spraying with DDT provided an effective measure to control malaria, which had been the main obstacle to colonization of the Dry Zone in modern times.[55] Irrigation development became linked to the nationalist vision of re-colonizing the Dry Zone with Sinhala peasants who were identified as "first inhabitants" of the island and were to be distinguished from Indian Tamil plantation workers brought in from the neighboring Madras Presidency during the era of British colonialism.[56] Ceylon's Sinhala elite aimed at "restoring the ancient glory of the hydraulic civilization that had been identified as the lost heritage of the Sinhala-Buddhist ethnic majority."[57] Yet irrigation (re)development and peasant colonization brought new human-made vector-breeding sites and peasant colonization settled some additional 253,000 Sinhala families in the impoverished Dry Zone, bringing ever more people in contact with vectors.[58] The developmental rearrangement of natural and social environments, driven by Sinhala nationalism, concludes Silva, was "at least partly responsible for the resurgence of malaria in Sri Lanka since 1967."[59] By 1982, malaria morbidity was back to the levels of the pre-DDT era.[60] Vector resistance to DDT was discovered in 1969 in Sri Lanka, antimalarial resistance among malaria parasites (chloroquine-resistant falciparum) in 1984, and multidrug-resistant falciparum malaria expanded in the following years.[61] Even the Civil War-induced malaria outbreak of 1990–2002 "had its antecedents in the ethno-nationalistically propelled development push of the Sri Lankan state."[62]

Despite their politically and economically close connections to this immediate big island neighbor to the northeast and being a part of the British Empire, the Maldives with their pronounced feverish history did not benefit from anti-malaria measures comparable to those pursued in Ceylon. The Maldives' program, by contrast, started at a time of malaria-related geopolitical disillusions in the mid-sixties. The eradication campaigns in other SEARO countries had already reached their zenith of success since the WHO's technocentric "magic bullets" approach, and thus the feasibility of eliminating malaria from the world as a public health problem had reached its limits.[63] From the mid-1950s *Anopheles* mosquitoes increasingly became resistant to DDT and with Rachel Carson's startling publication

Silent Spring in 1963, spraying campaigns were contested and the availability of DDT through the US declined.[64] When Sri Lanka faced a massive resurgence of malaria from the mid-1960s, the Maldivian eradication effort just had taken off.

An Eradication Program on the Move in the Maldives

The Maldives' Malaria Eradication Program comprised blood testing, mass drug administration, searching for mosquito larvae and plasmodium-infected mosquitoes, restricting potential mosquito breeding sites, and spraying DDT in all houses and roofed structures in inhabited and uninhabited islands. Mohammed Ismail Fulhu[65] joined the team after all houses in the capital Malé had been sprayed and the program was rolled out to the atolls in the late 1960s. He was born in 1948 and raised in Lhaviyani Atoll, 140 km north of Malé and started his career as a Domiciliary Health Worker with the WHO in malaria-control activities. Over more than 40 years he worked his way up the career ladder in the national health sector and in atoll politics. He has authored award-winning books on health developments in the Maldives.[66]

The eradication activities of the team of international WHO experts and trained locals were widely appreciated by the island communities, remembers Mr. Fulhu. The spacious hospital vessel *Golden Ray,* an outcome of development cooperation with the British, carried the team and all necessary equipment through the archipelago. It stopped at each island long enough to make sure that all islanders received the malaria medication chloroquine and promiquine for 5 consecutive days.[67] Mr. Fulhu estimates that one in three islanders was infected with malaria at the time. Islanders still acknowledged the malady by the Dhivehi (Maldivian) term *Heekaruvaafa anna hun,* indicating a fever (*hun*) that follows shivering. Children and teenagers were hit the hardest.

Mr. Fulhu remembers compliant island communities taking over crucial parts of the operation. The transfer of staff and equipment from *Golden Ray* to shore, for example, was usually by small rowing boats since most islands did not have any port or harbor at that time. The members of ten to twenty households per day had to remove all belongings for DDT spraying and could not return to their homes for one hour. In the early days of the program, writes Abdul Sattar Yoosuf in a fictional yet fact-based book on the experiences of the first cohort of community health workers in the Maldives, DDT:

"was of incessant use and whole islands would smell of it for days. The houses, many of them with coconut thatch partitions for walls, would have the marks of the white droplets dried on these and undersides of the roofs and even on whatever furniture they had. They were all covered with the familiar white marks left when the droplets dried. Keeping this residue was recommended as it would protect the insides of houses from the mosquito resting inside."[68]

Local community health workers, Island Chiefs, and spray-men were trained in the detection, treatment, and follow-up care of malaria patients as well as in vector-control activities. The inclusion of trained locals and a mobile eradication team were two crucial aspects in fruitfully localizing a global health policy to the specific conditions and challenges of an archipelago with a small dispersed population and a weak infrastructure. "Islandness," comprising geographical segmentation and island identity, turned out to be another crucial aspect conducive to sustained malaria eradication efforts in the Maldives. The small island communities were separated yet intensively connected by boat traffic. Movement from and to these islands was well defined and controllable. Boats coming to Malé from the islands, for example, were checked for the presence of mosquitoes and for larvae in stored water—if not, all the water they carried was emptied before entering Malé harbor—and all people entering Malé had to provide blood samples.[69] The island communities were sufficiently small to implement systematic blood testing and drug administration to allow outbreaks to be quickly recognized and treated, and for a rapid flow of risk-prevention communication. These qualities of islanders in epidemic times proved not only beneficial in finally defeating Maldive fever but also in the COVID-19 pandemic, as I have argued in more detail elsewhere.[70]

By 1974 the malaria-transmitting *Anopheles* mosquito species *A. tesselatus* and *A. subpictus* had almost disappeared. Around that time, in a kind of interlocking counter-development to the declining malaria cases, the first tourists arrived, which prepared the foundation for the future economic backbone of the island nation. The last indigenous infection with *Plasmodium falciparum* was recorded in 1975 in Haa-Alif Atoll. By 1979, family health workers took over malaria program duties from the Island Chiefs. In September 1984 the last more benign *P. vivax* case and thus the last indigenous case of malaria in the Maldives was reported in Baa Atoll.[71] Over the next decades, after overcoming Maldive fever, the island nation developed from one of the poorest, most remote and least developed countries in the world to one of South Asia's most affluent nations.[72] The risk of malaria being reintroduced, however, is looming and it thus remains a notifiable disease: case and vector surveillance as well as larva control continue to this day.[73]

Causal Factors for a Belated Success Story

This brings us back to the question of why the Maldives, with their distinct fever history, had not been on the radar of anti-malarial engagement much earlier, both by the colonial power and the subsequent global health endeavors. Compared with the exploitative plantation economy in Ceylon, the tiny sandy coral islands of the Maldives and a small, sea-foraging population admittedly had little to offer for colonial exploitation. In turn, Maldives' rulers were to an extent reluctant to accept foreign aid, assumes Mr. Fulhu, because British activities during the war and in the early post-war years had already interfered with the Maldives' independence in several unwelcome ways, as the following vignette demonstrates.

The southern atolls of the Maldives are geographically separated from the central parts of the archipelago by three mighty channels. The existence of a distinct southern dialect of Dhivehi (Maldivian) gives an idea of the challenges for the Malé rulers to reach and control these remote parts in the era of sail boats. The British military infrastructure in Gan brought prosperity to the south and the availability of western medicine and jobs contributed to a long-lasting antagonism between the central power and the southern periphery by enhancing it. Malé then tried to restrict free movement and direct trade between the southern atolls and Ceylon and between the military base in Gan and the locals. In reaction to these processes, the three atolls Addu, Fuvahmulah, and Huvadhoo broke away from the sovereign authority of the Sultan of the Maldives and formed the sovereign United Suvadive Republic on March 13, 1959.[74] Local voices often accuse the British of having "condoned local divisive sentiments until it rose to a crescendo."[75]

Abdulla Afeef Didi became the president of the short-lived separatist republic. Born in 1916 into a wealthy and influential Maldivian family of the south and educated in Egypt, the multi-lingual Afeef had served as liaison officer between the British and the locals since the mid-1950s. After the collapse of the secessionist republic, British authorities secretly deported Afeef from Maldivian territory in the fall of 1963. This was bypassing what Maldivians continue to see as falling under the jurisdiction of their government, which led to a fierce anti-British revolt.

On July 26, 1965, the Maldives gained independence. An accompanying agreement with the Maldivian government, however, allowed the RAF to continue using Gan Island as a staging post on the Far East run. During the late 1950s and the 1960s Gan was hence extensively used by RAF bombers, fighters, and transporters on their way to Singapore and other destinations in East Asia.

By 1970, however, the United Kingdom was withdrawing from its commitments east of the Suez. When the RAF Far East Air Force was disbanded in 1971, the major rationale for Gan Island as a British-controlled airstrip was fading. RAF Gan, nevertheless, remained in less frequent usage until 1975, when the geopolitical interests of the UK and the US (also in view of new aircraft technologies, but also of the end of wars in Vietnam and Laos) shifted to Diego Garcia in the Chagos archipelago some 750 km south of Gan.[76] The ongoing dispute over the maritime borders and the respective exclusive economic zones (EEZ) between the two neighboring archipelagos, however, still entangles the Maldives in the long breath of continuing decolonization struggles between the Chagossian islanders, Mauritius, and the UK.[77] Parallel to but independent of these late colonial and decolonizing processes as contexts for Maldivian health history, the Maldives are also intertwined in today's intensifying geopolitical rivalry between India and China in the Indian Ocean.

When the RAF staging post closed down on March 29, 1976 and Gan Island was handed back to full Maldivian Government authority, British geopolitical entanglements in local health developments once again became an issue. In a scandalizing tabloid article, journalist Iain Walker complains that by this withdrawal Britain abandoned 17,000 people "deprived of food and medical aid," since the last two British doctors also left in January 1976.[78]

So, we can identify delayed processes of decolonization affecting the Maldives, which gained independence in 1965, 17 years after Sri Lanka, while housing a British air base for another 11 years. This left traces on the local socio-political fabric, especially regarding the long history of tense relations between the sovereign in Malé and the south of the archipelago. For global health initiatives, in turn, the Maldives' small population represented comparatively insignificant case numbers. When 1.7 million malaria infections were registered in Sri Lanka in 1944,[79] the total population of the Maldives was about 80,000 (82,068 in 1946).[80] Finally, epidemiological and developmental rationales in the geopolitics of health may also have played a role in the Maldives' belated start to malaria eradication—a holoendemic and geographically challenging yet infrastructure-weak multi-island world. Under stable tropical conditions for intense, nearly year-round malaria transmission and high frequencies of inoculation (holoendemic conditions), "individuals developed resistance to the disease-causing blood stages of the malaria parasite." That immunity does indeed limit the disease's severity among adults.[81] Even the exclusion of the whole continent of Africa from the "global" malaria eradication program was justified by reference to insufficient infrastructure to carry out operations in rural areas, as well as by the (bewildering) assumption that there was no great urgency for an eradication program in this exceptionally intense malaria-transmission area.[82]

Conclusions: Island Models for the Region and Beyond

In line with their long health-related history, islands also served as natural laboratories in the anti-malarial campaigns in the SEARO region and provided landmark lessons for international health programs. Within the present volume's main theme, the case studies of the two South Asian Island states namely the Maldives and Sri Lanka contribute island viewpoints to the regional perspective on pandemics and geopolitics of health as proposed by Neelakantan.[83] Ecology, colonial dis/interest, war logistics and ideologies, as well as international health initiatives have had crucial impacts on both island settings. This concerns the perception of malaria as a problem and how to combat it, in relation to nation-building and public health development processes. Where Sri Lanka pioneered, however, Maldives was a latecomer. Subject to an extractive plantation economy since the early nineteenth century, Ceylon, on the contrary, served as a laboratory and model region for colonial anti-malarial interventions. The Sri Lankan case demonstrates that the proverbial magic bullet can have spectacular results but often fail to provide enduring answers.

The post-colonial "malaria blocks development discourse" matches the seasonality of farming. In Sri Lanka's Dry Zone, where the annual peak of the cultivation season coincides with enhanced vector breeding and malaria transmission during the rainy season, work days lost to sickness cause chronic poverty among peasants. In the Maldives, by contrast, the abundance of aquatic life and species of fish allow for fishing almost all year round. Unlike agriculture, fishing does not lead to a few critical work peaks (bottleneck periods) in the annual calendar upon which everything else depends.

Moreover, the colonial discourse about malaria as an obstacle to development and progress again became powerful and loaded with nationalist ideology as Sri Lanka gained independence in 1947. This resulted in a setback that brought infection rates back to pre-DDT levels in the early 1980s. In the Sri Lankan case, development did not ease but aggravated the malaria problem. Just a one-hour boat ride away, in the still fever-ridden Maldives, such a colonial medicine discourse was absent. The archipelago would not gain independence from Britain for another 17 years.

Sri Lanka is in line with and confirms the mainstream chronological sequence of the origins, rise, setback, and decline in the global malaria eradication effort. The Maldivian health trajectory, however, differed from these general currents of international health programs and global public health developments. Despite a pronounced feverish history, the Maldives were neglected in colonial anti-malarial discourses and left behind in the malaria eradication strategy that WHO SEARO had launched between 1957 and 1961 in the region. As causal factors for such an exceptional course of events in regional medical history this article suggests the delayed processes of decolonization, insignificant case numbers, and, eventually, a presumed immunity of the local population in this hyperendemic location shaped by environmental constraints.

The health of the general Maldivian population did not rank high on the colonizer's agenda, except for Addu atoll, where British forces came into close interaction with the potentially "infectious other." The eradication of malaria marks game-changing moments in Maldivian history. Since the mid-1970s, life-threatening fever attacks were relegated to the history books and the country opened up to international tourism. For the Maldives, malaria eradication was also an exercise in modernization and decolonizing health.

This chapter has examined this local Maldivian late colonial and early post-colonial history regarding malaria eradication in some detail. It has shown that the history of repelling febrile arthropod disease and its causative vectors in the Maldive islands has two distinctive phases of geopolitical embeddedness. The first phase was triggered by WWII logistics: geographically centered in the southern atolls, it marks the advent of western biomedicine in the colonial sultanate of the Maldives. Until the first biomedical center opened in 1948, the health facility in the RAF airbase in Addu atoll was an enclave of biomedical health services in the archipelago. In Ceylon, by contrast, triggered by the "national trauma" of the 1934/35 malaria epidemic, "a malaria control and health scheme covering the entire country was established (...) in 1937."[84] With some considerable delay, the second phase then put the Maldives on the global map of WHO's malaria eradication efforts: starting from the socio-political center Malé it covered the whole archipelago. This fell into the era of modernization and accompanied political developments toward the Republic of Maldives. With eradication programs for filariasis and malaria, the national health policy did develop in the Maldives but somewhat late, based on the WHO's standards reflecting "the Bandung spirit" that SEARO appropriated in their campaign against disease.[85]

In sum, the Maldives, as Asia's smallest country, succeeded in the campaign against filariasis and malaria where other ambitious global eradication plans had failed. For the WHO South-East Asia Region, as stated by the current SEARO Regional Director Poonam Khetrapal Singh, the Maldives' trajectory has shown "how eliminating a disease contributed to a nation's progress, and created a replicable model that is very relevant in other public health battles worldwide."[86] The Maldives' "historic achievements in public health"[87] thus provide a showcase which is belatedly reassuring some of the main pillars of the geopolitics of health in the post-WWII era. At least to an extent this rehabilitates the belief in the feasibility of the WHO's original action of "eliminating malaria from the world as a public health problem."[88] The Maldives' successful eradication affirms the focus on microbiological–immunological aspects of malaria transmission and health interventions aimed at interrupting the disease—a focus that was privileged in the South Asian geopolitics of health since the final years of colonial rule.

With a trajectory from feverish poverty to touristic affluence, the eradication of malaria in the Maldives demonstrates the successful localization of an international health initiative, or a substantial accomplishment in glocalization. Scale mattered in many regards in the Maldives' success story from the South Asian margins, ranging from seemingly insignificant, small case numbers to quarantine of a small island ground and tiny island communities.

This might be described as a maverick health trajectory path; as an exception to the rule: skipping colonial medicine at the margins of geography and colonial attention, followed by delayed decolonization and by the transformation from a wartime and post-war hub into a promising arena of public health for the local population.

Acknowledgments

This article is an outcome of a Canadian Social Sciences and Humanities Research Council partnership project on Indian Ocean World history, "Appraising Risk, Past and Present." I gratefully appreciate valuable suggestions by Andre Gingrich, Vivek Neelakantan, and the anonymous reviewers for improvement. I am pleased to acknowledge the substantial support and assistance Mr. Mohammed Ismail Fulhu, Aishath Shifneez Shakir, and my local interlocutors have been providing for my present research endeavor.

Notes

1 Randall M. Packard, *The Making of a Tropical Disease: A Short History of Malaria* (Baltimore: The Johns Hopkins University Press, 2007).
2 Bogdan C. Iacob, "Malariology and Decolonization: Eastern European Experts from the League of Nations to the World Health Organization," *Journal of Global History* (2022): 2. doi:10.1017/S1740022822000067.
3 Ibid.
4 Randall M. Packard, *A History of Global Health: Interventions into the Lives of Other Peoples* (Baltimore: The Johns Hopkins University Press 2016), 165.
5 David Arnold, "The Indian Ocean as a Disease Zone, 1500–1950," *South Asia: Journal of South Asian Studies* 14, no. 2 (1991): 4–21.
6 See also Regional Committee, "Study on Regionalization," Ninth Session Provisional Agenda Item 12, August 9, 1956, Doc SEA/RC9/10, WHO Library, Geneva (henceforth WHOL).
7 M. O. T. Iyengar, "Filariasis in the Maldive Islands," *Bulletin of the World Health Organization* 7 (1952): 375–403.
8 Ibid., 381.
9 Socrates Litsios, "The World Health Organization's Changing Goals and Expectations Concerning Malaria, 1948–2019." *História, Ciências, Saúde – Manguinhos* v.27, supl., set. (2020): 145–64, 150. doi:10.1590/S0104-59702020000300008.
10 Marcos Cueto, *Cold War, Deadly Fevers: Malaria Eradication in Mexico, 1955–1975* (Washington, DC and Baltimore: Woodrow Wilson Center Press and The Johns Hopkins University Press, 2007), 67.
11 See, for example, Sunil Amrith, *Decolonizing International Health: India and Southeast Asia, 1930–65* (Basingstoke: Palgrave MacMillan, 2006); Cueto, *Cold War, Deadly Fevers*; Packard, *The Making of a Tropical Disease*; Vivek Neelakantan, "The Campaign against the Big Four Endemic Diseases and Indonesia's Engagement with the WHO During the Cold War 1950s," in *Public Health and National Reconstruction in Post-War Asia: International Influences, Local* Transformations, Liping Bu edited (Abingdon, Oxon: Routledge, 2014), 154–74; Vivek Neelakantan, *Science, Public Health and Nation-Building in Soekarno-Era Indonesia* (Newcastle: Cambridge Scholars Publishing, 2017), 92–141; Sheila Zurbrigg, *Malaria in Colonial South Asia: Uncoupling Disease and Destitution* (London: Routledge India, 2019).
12 Packard, *The Making of a Tropical Disease*, 173.
13 Litsios, "The World Health Organization's Changing Goals," 154.

14 Amrith, *Decolonizing International Health*, 53.
15 Neelakantan, "The Campaign against the Big Four," 131.
16 Kalinga Tudor Silva, *Decolonisation, Development and Disease: A Social History of Malaria in Sri Lanka* (Hyderabad: Orient BlackSwan, 2014), 2–5.
17 Peter J. Brown, "Malaria, Miseria, and Underpopulation in Sardinia: The 'Malaria Blocks Development' Cultural Model," *Medical Anthropology* 17 (1997): 239–54. doi:10.1080/01459740.1997.9966139; Silva *Decolonisation, Development and Disease*, 130–32.
18 World Health Organization. Regional Office for South-East Asia, *Collaboration in Health Development in South-East Asia, 1948*–1988, SEARO Regional Publication no. 19 (New Delhi: SEARO, 1992), 131.
19 Lars Vilgon, "1344. Ibn Battuta," in *Maldive Odd History, Volume I: A Collection of 44 Entries Translated and Transliterated into English from 11 Languages*, Lars Vilgon edited (Malé: National Centre for Linguistic and Historical Research, 2001), 41.
20 François Pyrard, *The Voyage of Franiçois Pyrard of Laval to the Bast Indies, the Maldives, the Moluccas, and Brazil*, trans. and edited with notes by Albert Gray, assisted by H.C.P. Bell from the 3rd French edition of 1619, Vol. 1 (New York: Burt Franklin Publisher, 1887), 82–85.
21 Remco Raben, "European Periphery at the Heart of the Ocean: The Maldives, 17th–18th Centuries," in *International Conference on Shipping, Factories and Colonization (Brussels, 24–26 November 1994)*, John Everaert and J. Parmentier edited (Collectanea maritima Vol. 7. Brussels: Academie Royale des Sciences d'Outre-Mer, 1996), 51.
22 H. C. P. Bell, *The Maldive Islands: Monograph on the History, Archaeology and Epigraphy* (Malé: Novelty Printers and Publishers, 2002 [1940]), 6.
23 Ibid., 14.
24 E.g. Clarence Maloney, *People of the Maldive Islands* (New Delhi: Orient Longman, 1980), 127, 398–99. See also SEARO, *0 Malaria-Free Maldives* (New Delhi: SEARO, 2016).
25 Mr. Ismail (a pseudonym) in electronic discussion with the author, September 30, 2021, in English and Dhivehi, conveyed and in parts translated by Aishath Shifneez Shakir.
26 Packard, *The Making of a Tropical Disease*, 19–25.
27 Eva-Maria Knoll, "The Maldives as an Indian Ocean Crossroads," in *Oxford Research Encyclopedia of Asian History*, Edward Alpers et al. edited (New York: Oxford University Press). https://oxfordre.com/asianhistory/view/10.1093/acrefore/9780190277727.001.0001/acrefore-9780190277727-e-327
28 M. O. T. Iyengar, M. I. Mathew, and M. A. U. Menon, "Malaria in the Maldive Islands," *Indian Journal of Malariology* 7, no. 1 (1953): 1–3. M. O. T. Iyengar and M. A. U. Menon, "Mosquitoes of the Maldive Islands," *Bulletin of Entomological Research* 46 (1955): 1–10.
29 J. R. M. Schepens, "Malaria Control in the Maldives" *WHO Consultant Assignment Report, October 1974–July 1980*, World Health Organization Project MAV MPD 001.
30 World Health Organization, *0. Malaria-Free Maldives*, 7.
31 World Health Organization, *Collaboration in Health Development*, 128.
32 Jack L. S. Coulter, *The Royal Naval Medical Service* Administration, vol. 1 (London: Her Majesty's Stationery Office, 1954), 218–20.
33 M. Lewis, D. Michael, Abdul Azeez Yousuf, Kriangkrai Lerdthusnee, Ahmed Razee, Kirkvitch Chandranoi and James W. Jones, "Scrub Typhus Reemergence in the Maldives," *Emerging Infectious Diseases* 9, no. 12 (2003): 1638, doi:10.3201/eid0912.030212.

34 Chakraborty, Sayantani, and Nilendu Sarma, "Scrub Typhus: An Emerging Threat", *Indian Journal of Dermatology* 62, no. 5 (2017): 278. doi: 10.4103/ijd. IJD_388_17: 10.4103/ijd.IJD_388_17.
35 Lewis, Michael, Yousuf et al., "Scrub Typhus Reemergence", 1639.
36 Allen L. Richard and Ju Jiang, "Scrub Typhus: Historic Perspective and Current Status of the Worldwide Presence of *Orientia* Species," *Tropical Medicine and Infectious Disease* 2020 5, no. (2020): 1–8. In the Maldives scrub typhus re-emerged 58 years after the WWII cases, again with a focus in the southern atolls, with an outbreak with 168 cases and 10 deaths in 2002. The disease mostly affected agricultural laborers and migrant workers on tourist resorts. Refer Lewis, Michael, Yousuf et al., "Scrub Typhus Reemergence," 1638. Scrub typhus remains a public health problem in contemporary Maldives with some 50 to 70 cases annually. See Stephen Berger, *Infectious Diseases of the Maldives* (Gideon E-Book Series. Los Angeles: Gideon Informatics, 2020), 231.
37 *The Royal Naval Medical Service. Volume II. Operations.* By Coulter, Jack L. S. (London: Her Majesty's Stationary Office, 1956), 140–42.
38 Iyengar, "Filariasis," 375–403. Iyengar and Menon, "Mosquitoes of the Maldive". Iyengar and Menon, "Malaria in the Maldive". Compare Mohammed Ismail Fulhu, *Health Care in Maldives Yesterday and Past* (Republic of Maldives: Print-N-Gard (Pvt) Ltd., (2014 [2010]), 172–78.
39 Nicolas Wright, and Keith Morris, "The RAF's Loneliest Outpost," *The Illustrated London News* 6856, no. 257 (1970), 15.
40 In 1942 the RAF also had a second local presence on Hithadhoo, another island in southern Addu Atoll. Complementary to the southern RAF Gan presence, there was also a short-lived British base at the northern tip of the Maldives. According to former Island Chief Abdulla Waheed, the staging post in Kelaa, located at the northeastern fringe of the archipelago, was used for 11 months in 1945 as a refueling station for war planes, run by around 100 RAF military staff and around 400 workers ("Kelaa in the Time of British," IDEAS – Island Development and Environmental Awareness Society, https:// ideaskelaa.wordpress.com/2017/07/23/kelaa-in-the-time-of-british/.)
41 cf. Rohan Deb Roy and Guy N.A. Attewell, ed., *Locating the Medical: Explorations in South Asian History.* (New Delhi: Oxford University Press, 2018).
42 Wright and Morris, "The RAF's Loneliest," 17.
43 Royal Naval Medical Service Vol. II, 140.
44 Ibid. Vol. I, 219. The spleen occupied a prominent space in theories of malaria-specific immunity and the colonial normative view of native South Asian bodies as afflicted by climate. Splenic pathology, especially enlargement ("tropical splenomegaly") indicated chronic suffering from malaria among other diseases (Sudipta Sen, "Confessions of the Unfriendly Spleen: Medicine, Violence, and That Mysterious Organ of Colonial India," in *Locating the Medical: Explorations in South Asian History,* Rohan Deb Roy and Guy N. A. Attewell edited (New Delhi: Oxford University Press, 2018), 82.
45 Royal Naval Medical Service Vol. II, 140.
46 Ibid., 141–42.
47 Fulhu, *Health Care Maldives,* 27. A Sri Lankan doctor of Tamil descent, employed by the Maldivian Government, practiced since June 1931 in Malé (Fulhu, *Health Care Maldives,* 71).
48 *Statistical Year Book of the Maldives*, Table 3.1. (Malé : National National Bureau of Statistics).
49 Silva, *Decolonisation, Development and Disease*, 9–13, 154.
50 Ibid., 14.

51   Margaret Jones. *Striving for Equity: Healthcare in Sri Lanka from Independence to the Millennium, 1948–2000* (Hyderabad (IN): Orient Blackswan, 2020), 5.

52   Silva, *Decolonisation, Development and Disease*, 135–36.

53   Kalinga Tudor Silva, "'Public Health' for Whose Benefit? Multiple Discourses on Malaria in Sri Lanka," *Medical Anthropology* 17, no. 3 (1997): 199–200, 195–214. http://dx.doi.org/10.1080/01459740.1997.9966137.

54   Silva, *Decolonisation, Development and Disease*, 133–58.

55   Ibid., 137–41.

56   Ibid., 138.

57   Ibid., 132–34. In Sri Lanka malaria had been foremost a problem of the Dry Zone, which had been the center of the ancient hydraulic civilization, which reached its peak around the 12th century CE. This formerly rich cultivated land had turned into a semi-jungle with neglected tanks remaining from the ancient elaborate irrigation system in addition to the "communally maintained local reservoirs (tanks)" of each peasant village community. The "possible role [of malaria] in the fall of the ancient hydraulic civilization (...) is subject to speculation" (Kalinga Tudor Silva, "Ayurveda, Malaria and the Indigenous Herbal Tradition in Sri Lanka," *Social Science Medicine* 33, no. 2 (1991): 154–55).

58   Silva, *Decolonisation, Development and Disease*, 189.

59   Ibid., 142.

60   Ibid., 143–44.

61   Ibid., 151–52.

62   Ibid., 157.

63   Amrith, *Decolonizing International Health*, 18.

64   *World Health Organization. Collaboration in Health Development*, 130.

65   Mohammed Ismail Fulhu in electronic discussion with the author, September 30, 2021, in English and Dhivehi, conveyed and in parts translated by Aishath Shifneez Shakir.

66   E.g. Fulhu, *Health Care Maldives*.

67   For detailed descriptions of the medical launch *Golden Ray* see ibid., 153–54 and the Maldives Malaria Eradication Program pages 183–94.

68   Abdul Sattar Yoosuf, *Unsung Heroes: An Island Health Worker's Journey* (New Delhi: Amber Books, 2012), chap. 4, Kindle. See also his newsletter article Abdul Sattar Yoosuf, "Eliminating Malaria in Maldives," *Health in South-East Asia. SEARO Newsletter* 7, no. 1 (2014): 8–10.

69   Fulhu, *Health Care Maldives,* 185–86.

70   Eva-Maria Knoll, "How the Maldives Have Navigated Disease and Development," *Current History* 120, no. 825 (2021): 153–55, DOI: https://doi.org/10.1525/curh.2021.120.825.152.

71   *World Health Organization, 0. Malaria-Free Maldives*, 11.

72   Malaria eradication revealed a correlation between the historic malaria prevalence in the atolls and a high prevalence of beta-thalassaemia in the country, a gene variant providing some protection against *Falciparum* malaria (Firdous, Naila, Stephen Gibbons and Bernadette Modell, "Falling Prevalence of Beta-thalassaemia and Eradication of Malaria in the Maldives," *Journal of Community Genetics* 2 (2011): 176–77. doi:10.1007/s12687-011-0054-0.) The risk of both parents carrying the beta-thalassaemia trait (a selective advantage deriving from a feverish past) and passing it on to the next generation persists as a major public health issue in the Maldives (Eva-Maria Knoll, "Inherited Without History? Maldive Fever and its Aftermath," in *Disease Dispersion and Impact in the Indian Ocean World*, Gwyn Campbell and Eva-Maria Knoll edited (Cham: Palgrave Macmillan, 2020), 255–84.

73 "Malaria on the Decline in WHO South-East Asia Region; Efforts Must Continue as Risks Persist," World Health Organization News Release SEAR/PR/1721, December 4, 2019, https://www.who.int/southeastasia/news/detail/04-12-2019-malaria-on-the-decline-in-who-south-east-asia-region-efforts-must-continue-as-risks-persist-who.

74 James Minahan, "Suvadivians: Huvadu," in *Encyclopedia of the Stateless Nations: Ethnic and National Groups around the World*, vol. 4, *S–Z*. (Westport, CT: Greenwood, 2002), 1799–1802.

75 Yoosuf, *Unsung Heroes,* chap. 3.

76 "Unit History: RAF Gan," Forces War Records, accessed August 7, 2018. https://www.forces-war-records.co.uk/units/4098/raf-gan.

77 Cf. David Vine, *Island of Shame: The Secret History of the U.S. Military Base on Diego Garcia* (Princeton: Princeton University Press, 2009).

78 Walker secretly visited Addu Atoll together with photographer Roger Bamber to document the situation one year after RAF's pull-out. See Iain Walker, "Paradise Lost: I see Britain's Shame – the People we Have Abandoned to a Living Death," *The Sun*, May 16, 1977.

79 Silva, *Decolonisation, Development and Disease*, 136.

80 National Bureau of Statistics. *Statistical Yearbook of Maldives 2019*, Table 3.1.

81 Packard, *Making of a Tropical Disease, 28–29*. On the significance of differences in malaria susceptibility and acquired immunity in the geopolitics of health see Zurbrigg, *Malaria in Colonial South Asia,* chap. 1–2.

82 Elizabeth Fee, Marcos Cueto and Theodore Brown, "At the Root of the World Health Organization's Challenges: Politics and Regionalization," *American Journal of Public Health* 106, no. 11 (April 2016): 1916.

83 Vivek Neelakantan, "History of Pandemics in Southeast Asia: A Return of National Anxieties," *ISIS Current Bibliography* (2021), https://isiscb.org/2020/pandemics-in-south-east-asia/, accepted. See also "Introduction," this volume.

84 Silva, *Decolonisation, Development and Disease*, 18, 135.

85 Neelakantan, "The Campaign against the Big Four," 132.

86 *World Health Organization. Regional Office for South-East Asia A Nation Shows the Way: Elimination of Malaria in Maldives* (New Delhi: SEARO, 2016), 1, https://apps.who.int/iris/handle/10665/251840.

87 World Health Organization Country Office for Maldives, *Maldives: A Journey of Health* (Geneva: WHO, 2017), 42, https://apps.who.int/iris/handle/10665/259178.

88 *World Health Organization. Regional Office for South-East Asia. Collaboration in Health Development,* 130.

4 Thailand's Rural Doctor Society in the 1970s–80s and Its Struggles to Improve Health in the Countryside

Davisakd Puaksom

Introduction

This is the time that lives have fallen off like leaves of the tropical deciduous forest in the dry season. At this moment, when Hades rules his necropolis over the living world, the COVID-19 pandemic has proven once again that citizenship in Thailand is meaningless without legal protection, literally as dust under the sovereign's feet, as their respectful pronoun in addressing the king puts it.[1] Practically, the medicalizing state in Thailand and the worldwide movement toward universal health coverage that had become a great success of populist politics during the early 2000s has been faced with a new viral challenge.[2] As a legacy of a populist government, this health scheme would have been abolished over the years by successive military juntas since the royal sanctioned coup in 2014, had it not been an efficient and beneficial policy for the public health of the nation. Nonetheless, the pandemic challenge has called for a review of Thailand's health system and its health care reforms in recent decades.

The most conspicuous political change in Thailand—following the conclusion of the Cold War in 1991—was not the country's trajectory toward democratization but the movement for primary health care.[3] Not quite unlike the Barefoot Doctors in China's rural medical program during the 1960s, an influential factor in Thailand's health care reforms during the past decades was the rural doctor movement.[4] Rural healthcare provisions in other Southeast Asian countries were characterized as intervention of the postcolonial state: for example, Indonesia's Bandung Plan of the 1950s that aimed to realize an equitable distribution of health care between urban and rural areas.[5] By contrast, the Philippines pioneered voluntary healthcare engagement that involved NGOs.[6] Thailand's rural doctor movement was neither state-driven nor a voluntary healthcare engagement that mobilized NGOs but a professional coalition that aimed to redress the urban bias of the Thai health system. Although few publications have focused on the successes and failures of Thai health care reforms,[7] the active engagement of the Rural Doctor Society has scarcely been examined by medical historians.[8]

DOI: 10.4324/9781003332060-5

Conventional historiography depicts the establishment of the Rural Doctor Society as inspired by the WHO's Declaration on Primary Healthcare at Alma Ata (1978).[9] Nevertheless, it cannot be denied that a combination of domestic pressures and foreign influences led to the founding of the Rural Doctor Society in 1976. These included: (a) the early political awakening of Thai medical professionals since their college years during the late 1960s; (b) the World Health Assembly (WHA) 1976 resolution urging member states to develop Primary Health Care programs; and (c) the WHO's advocacy of the Chinese Barefoot Doctor model for the health systems of developing countries by the mid-1970s.[10]

Because the study heavily relied on in-depth interviews, Joseph Harris' brief explanation of the growth of the Society was out of date and focused solely on important individuals associated with the health care reform.[11] None of the historical studies have illustrated a full development of the Rural Doctor Society since its inception, and inscription within the Society's publications during the late 1970s and 1980s before its movement had formed the invisible college called the Sampran Group, an unofficial think-tank. By the early-2000s, the Group influenced Thailand's movement toward Universal Health Coverage. But the country's movement toward universal coverage merits a separate article.

The Abortive Beginning of the Rural Doctor Federation

Conceived in the mid-1970s, the Rural Doctor Society was arguably a product of historical conditions largely formulated earlier with US technical assistance in building up provincial hospitals throughout the country in the 1950s, in exchange for Thailand's support of the US containment policy in Asia. In the heat of the cold war, the US psychological and military strategy teamed up with Thailand's military junta in encountering the communist movement. The US heavily invested in Thailand's Accelerated Rural Development Agency since the late 1950s, including provincial hygiene, mobile medical services, and in an inchoate primary health care project in Phitsanulok between 1966 and 1968.[12] In parallel with these developments, the regional universities were founded in the early 1960s, partially with funding from the Rockefeller Foundation, in order to train medical practitioners who would strengthen the force of the free world in the rural areas that were prone to communist infiltration.

The Social Science Association of Thailand (SSAT) was also founded in March 1956 to countervail the growing force of leftist intellectuals. In 1957, a large number of leftist intellectuals and journalists were incarcerated without trial after the military junta led by Field Marshal Sarit Thanarat seized power.[13] A few years after the coup, a rather critical journal, *Sangkhomsat Parithat* [Social Science Review], began publication in 1963, under the SSAT with financial assistance from the Asia Foundation and edited by Sulak Sivaraksa, the progressive royalist and the Lampeter graduate. As it turned

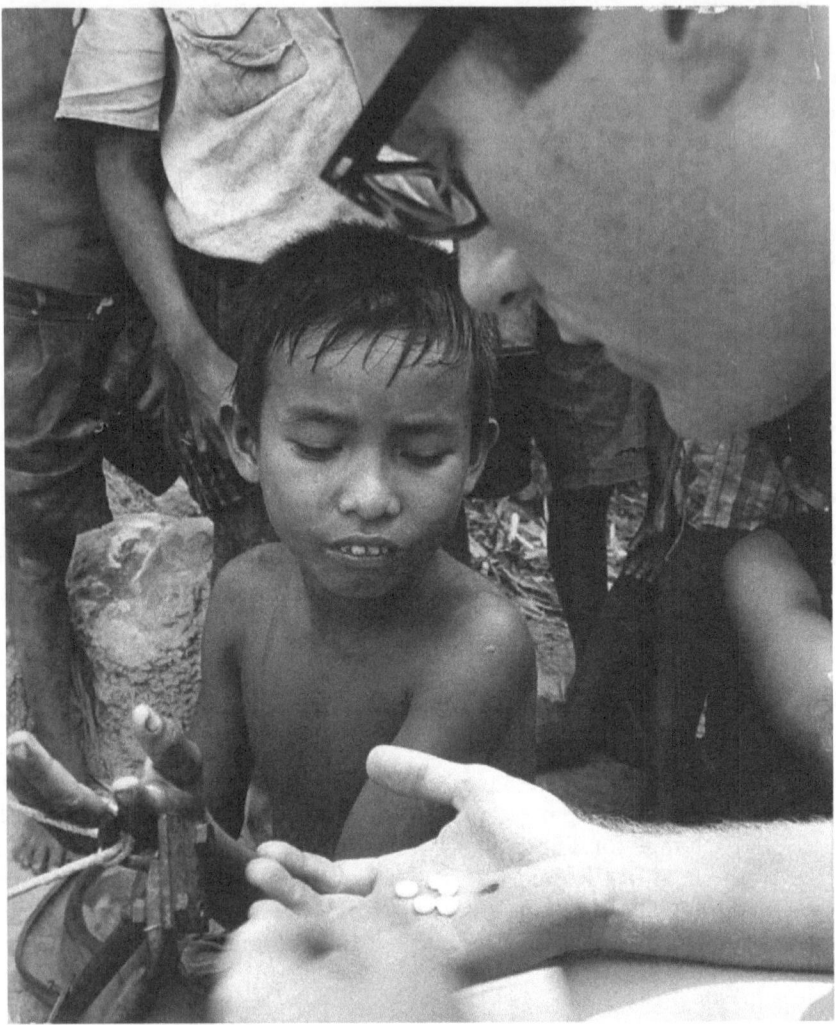

Figure 4.1 Peace Corps Volunteer John Tucker, working in the AID-sponsored
malaria eradication program, dispensing anti-malarial pills at a village
near Nam Pong, Thailand (1968).

Peace Corps Volunteer John Tucker, working in the AID-sponsored malaria eradication program, dispenses malaria pills in a village near Nam Pong, Thailand, 1968
Photo   Credit: USAID/Carl   Purcell;   https://www.flickr.com/photos/usaidasia/albums/
72157627506230488

out, the journal became a public forum of social critique and attracted
attention from the conservatives and the liberals alike. To encourage university students' engagement, Sulak invited a few medical students, particularly Vichai Chokevivat, to have their own voices in the student-led journal's
regular special issues between March 1966 and July 1971.[14]

Apparently, Sulak's initiative not only provided a forum for thoughts and discussions among the university students and social activists but subtly stirred the political awakening of the young generation. Soon after, the government enacted a conscription policy that mandated that medical students serve in the health center for 6 years subsequent to their graduation. The mandatory conscription of newly minted medical graduates to work in rural areas was intended to redress the acute shortage of physicians across Thailand and the inequitable distribution of physicians, mostly concentrated in urban areas such as Bangkok, and to halt a massive migration of medical graduates to the US during the Vietnam War.[15]

Medical students quickly mobilized their organizations in an attempt to resist. Eventually, the cabinet passed a resolution on April 14, 1967, that the tuition fee of incoming medical students would be deferred to the third year. Third-year students had to pay the tuition fee set at 10,000 baht per annum. The resolution stipulated that not more than 25 percent of students had to pay fees. Those students who were exempted from paying tuition fees were considered grant recipients from the Thai government and had to serve in the civil service or military hospitals for three-years after their graduation.[16] Anyone who failed to comply with this regulation was fined three times the tuition fee. Thereafter, the committee, appointed by the cabinet on September 15, 1967, had stated that newly minted graduates had to spend 1 year of their internship in a place assigned by the Medical Council Board and had to sign a 2-year compulsory contract with the civil service or military hospitals. Three years later, on December 8, 1970, after the first cohort of these practitioners had been posted to their health care centers, the cabinet had the compensation changed and remuneration increased from 120,000 to 200,000 baht; and the remuneration doubled to 400,000 baht on 17 April 1973.[17]

The implementation of this 2-year conscription of state-sponsored medical students to work in rural areas created much discontent among medical students and the dissenting voices varied from resistance and non-cooperation to participation in conscription. Resistance against conscription gradually gained momentum. Disgruntled medical students from four medical schools: that is, Siriraj, Chulalongkorn, Ramathibodi, and Chiangmai, held a meeting at Chiangmai University between March 28 and 30, 1969. Eventually the Medical Students Center of Thailand (MSCT) was established to represent their voices to the Ministry of Public Health (MoPH).[18] Thereafter, these activist medical students established several more students' organizations such as the Mahidol Medical Students' Union and the Mahidol Students' Union which held their first demonstration in 1972 against the government's regulation that prevented female students from becoming civil servants and working in the rural areas.[19] During the mass student movement in October 1973, the MSCT and these organizations had also joined rank with the Students Center of Thailand (SCT) in mobilizing the masses to topple the military junta, especially in organizing emergency medical teams for the movement.[20]

The student movement in the mid-1970s temporarily brought down the decade-and-a-half-long military regime.[21] At the time, Manit Prapansin, Director of Health Care Center at Sri Chiangmai, Nongkhai, had experienced the harsh working conditions of medical interns. He took the lead in sending a circular letter to all rural health care centers in Thailand, calling for an assembly to review their situation. In his letter, Manit had convinced the MoPH to hold a convention at Khao-yai, Korat, a sanctuary in the northeast of Bangkok, on April 24 and 25, 1976, with a gathering of 50–60 rural practitioners. At the convention, prior to the ministry's program, rural healthcare workers held a meeting and declared that they would establish "The Rural Doctor Federation" (Sahaphan phaet chonnabot), which aimed to resolve public health problems in rural areas. In the second convention of the federation at Bangramung, Chonburi, between June 5 and 6, 1979, Prasop Phonphai (Bangpa-in hospital, Ayutthaya) was then elected as The Rural Doctor Federation's first official president and Manit was the secretary.[22]

In the only issue of the federation's journal *Warasan sahaphan phaet chonnabot* [*Journal of the Rural Doctor Federation*], published in August 1976, the members declared that the federation aimed to coordinate medical practitioners at the district level throughout the country in order to share experiences and opinions of their practices, to crystallize those experiences, and to support the public health policies that would truly benefit national interests. Moreover, the federation would provide an impetus in the delivery of health care to the rural areas of the country. The Rural Doctor Federation's objectives were as follows: (1) to study problems affecting access to healthcare in rural areas; (2) to share the experiences of physicians working in rural areas of Thailand and co-ordinate the relationship between members and related organizations; and (3) to encourage the medical practitioners to work in rural health care posts.[23]

The subsequent tragic events of the October 6, 1976 massacre when some students were shot at Thammasat University and a few others were hanged on a tamarind tree and burnt with tires by right-wing paramilitary groups, was decisive in restoring the ultra-royalists and the military regime to power.[24] Amidst a thorny political conflict, an army coup was staged against the elected government, with royal assent, claiming to restore the country's stability and to purge the communist insurgency. The hardline anti-communist law professor Thanin Kraivixian was picked to take charge as prime minister, announcing that he had a 20-year plan to implant the country's real democracy. The military junta had mobilized the entire state apparatus for the suppression of communism. The liberated areas of the Communist Party of Thailand (CPT), especially the mountainous ranges in the north, the northeast, and the south, thus benefitted from a massive influx of university students, left-leaning and liberal alike.[25]

On the very morning of the massacre, officials from the national security agency had swiftly arrested the suspected leftist alliances and social activists throughout the country. Vichai Chokevivat, by that time the director of the health care center at Payakphumpisa, Mahasarakham, was incarcerated without trial for 1 month before he was released with a condition that he had to be immediately transferred from that province. After the release, Vichai was moved to Nakhorn Phathom, an adjacent province of Bangkok. Manit Prapansin himself had paid a visit to Vichai in that very night and would have been arrested together with Vichai had he not left earlier that morning.[26]

Political activists considered as radical elements were targeted or licensed to be killed by the military or rightwing paramilitary throughout the country. Some were mysteriously shot, such as leaders of the Farmers and Peasants Federation, and several others experienced assassination attempts.[27] Many medical students and practitioners fled to join with the CPT's revolutionary force, including Prommin Lertsuridet (Ramathibodi University), Chaturon Chaisaeng (Chiangmai University), Phondet Pinpratheep (Mahidol University), and Virasak Chongsuvivatvong (Ramathibodi University).[28] Some of the CPT's allies, particularly Suriya Vongkhongkhathep, Pichate Leelaphanmetha, and Viroj Tangcharoensathien decided to remain in town as they had taken up private practice to support their colleagues' affiliation with the CPT's medical service in the jungle. A few students even paid short visits to the CPT bases, such as Viroj did in the south in 1979.[29] A few others were rumored to have helped by trafficking medical supplies to the CPT bases.

Conceived at a time of political turbulence in Thailand's modern history, the Rural Doctor Federation abruptly collapsed in just a few months after the meeting. After the October 1976 massacre, Manit resigned from the civil service to work instead with a private hospital at Korat. Fortunately, within 1 year in office, Thanin's government was overthrown by another coup, led by a more soft-line general, Kriangsak Chamanan, on October 20, 1977. Manit then returned to the government office at Prakhonechai hospital, Buriram Province. In December 1977, Manit coaxed Suwit Vibulphonprasert—a first-class honors graduate from Ramathibodi, who had just started his career at Bangruat, a community hospital. Suwit was urged to pay visits to the rural practitioners at the district health care centers in the northeast. All the practitioners whom Suwit visited supported the idea of reconvening the group. Later, they paid a visit to Anand Menaruji, the director of Banphai hospital, and urged him to contact Chalo Guptavindhu, then the deputy director of provincial public health office at Khonkhaen. In a private meeting, they asked Chalo to convene a meeting in which they would establish a medical society.[30]

Eventually, a meeting at Khosa hotel, Khonkhaen, was organized in February 1978, with 37 participants who were medical practitioners at the district level, mostly from the northeast. Apart from sharing their experiences and difficulties, the congregation unanimously agreed to rebuild the group, but its name was changed to the Rural Doctor Society (*chomrom phaet chonnabot*) in order to soften its political impact, with Uthain Jaranasri as its first president; Manit was once again its secretary, with Suwit as his deputy.[31]

Another Road to Alma Ata

Concomitant with the development of these practitioners' political awakening, a surge of rural health care in international Cold War politics was shaping the feature of Thailand's health care system. Especially as the Chinese Communist Revolution (1949) had offered another path of progress toward an industrialized and democratic society, health care and medicine in rural Thailand caused public disquiet. Thereafter, rural health care was a contentious arena of socialist propaganda. US international policymakers also co-opted a perspective that eradicating epidemic and endemic diseases would not only secure raw materials for its industrial production and provide markets for its commodities, but it would also be a measure of its world dominance and would further the containment of the communist insurgency.[32]

With a concern that the neglect of rural health and medicine would prove congenial to communist infiltration, US technical assistance and foreign aid flowed to developing countries to secure loyalty of their political elites. In the case of Thailand, a large proportion of US aid was assigned for the country's economic and infrastructure development, including the rural hygiene projects, mobile medical services, and primary health care projects.[33]

Earlier, the emphasis on a training of first-class physicians in biomedicine and the resistance to a training of practical health workers had largely dominated Thailand's medical education since the late 1920s when assistance to reform the medical school was provided by the Rockefeller Foundation.[34] Nevertheless, the insufficient numbers of physicians and inequitable distribution between the urban and rural areas called for other solutions such as a compulsory 2-year work requirement in rural health services and alternative paths of health care through preventive medicine that was cheaper in cost and covered larger numbers of the population served.

The necessity of primary health workers in ameliorating health conditions in the rural area became ever urgent, in 1968. At the time, China had officially launched its rural medical program under the directive of Chairman Mao.[35] Coincidentally, in that year the Ministry of Public Health had commenced another project on primary health care at Saraphi District, in Chiangmai Province, during 1968–71. Success of the Saraphi and other subsequent projects had led to the conclusion that health volunteers, traditional midwives, and medical technicians with basic training affiliated with the subdistrict health station would be the key measures in extending health care services to all rural populations.[36]

Eventually, rural health became a crisis that demanded structural adjustment within the Ministry of Public Health in the early 1970s. Political struggles had dragged on for years to integrate preventive medicine into the administrative structure and annual budget. Finally, by 1975, the Ministry of Health issued a decree to extend community hospitals to all district levels throughout the country, in which these freshly graduated physicians had to render their services.[37] Meanwhile, preventive medicine was a partial measure until the primary health care was instituted as another platform of health service in the fourth national plan for public health development in 1977, 1 year ahead of the Alma Ata declaration on primary health care in 1978.[38]

Government decrees in Thailand mandated the provision of rural healthcare; physicians affiliated with the Rural Doctor Society were among the most ardent advocates for this policy. The political awakening of local medical students in the late 1960s, the influence of the Barefoot Doctors Model from China, and the WHO's support for primary healthcare were among the national and international influences that contributed to this.

Rural Inscriptions

After its (re)founding in February 1978, the Rural Doctor Society decided to resume publishing its periodical, namely *Warasan chomrom phaetchonnabot* [Journal of the Rural Doctor Society], with its first issue in June 1978 edited by Santiphap Chaiyavongkiat, then affiliated with the Ratanaburi hospital in Surin Province.[39] On its first cover, there was a large picture of four mobile medical personnel operating their basic medical practice at a school. At the bottom, there was an announcement printed in big font that it was a forum for an exchange of ideas among the rural doctors throughout the country. Though it was unclear whether they were students, interns, or registered professionals, undoubtedly this picture captured a routine reality of medical practice these young physicians were facing in their upcountry health stations. The announcement thus carried an ideological rhetoric impregnated with certain romantic ideals of rural health work. In short, their profession was a charitable enterprise aimed to ameliorate the country's underdevelopment and redress the people's grievances.

On its very first page was a presidential address that contextualized the emergence of the Rural Doctor Society. Uthain Jaranasri related that in the gatherings of medical practitioners who served in the medical and hygienic centers (MHC) and community hospitals (CH) at the district level during the previous 5 years, there were repeated discussions about the impediments to their work. The challenges faced by these physicians could not be addressed by curative practice alone. Some practitioners had no desire to work at the district level or in remote areas due to poor remuneration. In 1976, a group of practitioners who served in the MHCs and CHs thus held a meeting and called themselves the Rural Doctors. They sought to address the impediments that prevented the expansion of health facilities to rural Thailand. Nevertheless, their movement was halted, since "the politics at that time" after the military coup in October 1976 did not allow the founding of groups or factions. According to Uthain, the small MHCs or CHs operated with a modest budget and limited medical personnel. But newly graduated and inexperienced practitioners were dispatched to serve in such workplaces without appropriate preparation. It was only those who had served or were serving in the MHCs or CHs who could understand, share experiences, and offer guidance with solutions for improvement that would overcome their impediments. They could be sympathetic with those who were perplexed. In early 1978, there was thus a re-restoration of the Society that aimed to be a medium for contemplating their problems.[40]

In the Society's regulation published in its first issue, its objectives were to study public health problems in rural areas and to search for solutions that would enable better medical service for the people. It stated clearly that the Society would not get involved with politics. The former members of the Rural Doctor Federation would automatically retain their membership and any medical practitioner could apply for membership for a 100-baht fee. General practitioners, residents, interns, or medical students could also apply for associate membership, but two recommendations from general members were needed along with a lower fee of 30 baht only.[41]

Understanding the rural conditions and its health problems was thus their prime agenda. Santiphap wrote in his first editorial foreword that the journal would publish experiences of those practitioners who had served in the district health centers or community hospitals, as well as letters to the Society in the form of queries or suggestions, academic articles useful to rural medicine, criticisms, and even proposals to improve one's own health center or hospital.[42] In in its first issue, apart from the presidential address, the journal published the new government's financial regulations, brief observations on the rural doctor's lives, short interviews with two practitioners from Buriram and Surin provinces, and content on the procedural delays encountered in the procurement of medical equipment.

Imbued by the spirit of the Alma Ata Declaration in 1978, rural health issues were featured in the Journal of the Rural Doctor Society. Petrichor or the pleasant earthy scent and "the provincial aura" of rural areas and shanty towns featured in the journal's pages.[43] Deficiency of medical equipment, budgets, pharmaceuticals, and staffing became regular if painful features that cut across the whole public health care system in rural areas.[44] In squatter accommodation, located at some distance from the urban areas, welfare housing was far below the usual standard; monsoonal floods and power shortages were not uncommon.[45]

Apparently, administrative bottlenecks were decisive here. At a few hospitals, requests to replace the hospital's electrical wiring would take months and practitioners faced charges of corruption.[46] The new director of the Sichon hospital was even greeted with flying bullets aimed at the police station just opposite to the hospital.[47] Another practitioner was allegedly reported by his superior to the counter-insurgency officer. As a suspected communist element, he was then followed by a security officer.[48] Few, if not many, experienced the corruption and abuse of resources they had expected.[49] And an empty office was not unusual.[50]

Rural health work was clearly articulated as a part and parcel of expanding modernization.[51] In other words, these physicians sought to transform rural Thailand. In Vichai Chokevivat's recollection of his early encounters, the northeasterner was a "walking" embodiment of the underdevelopment. He was a drunkard, an indolent, and a gambling addict. A village youngster would keep untidy long hair, wear jeans, and be unfriendly. It would take Vichai some time to discover the reasons deep behind such appearances. These people were poverty-stricken, he wrote, from the time they were embryos in their mothers' wombs:

> Once born, they were raised carelessly. They had to struggle with the hardships of everyday life, living from hand-to-mouth, since they were young. The kids raised cattle, and at various places he could see these children use a small casting net to catch fish or shrimp in a pond or help their parents to peel hemp from jute plants along the road. At night when it was raining, they would go out to catch some frogs so they could have a meal at school the next day, etcetera.[52]

The above quote succinctly illustrated that the rural Northeast of Thailand was underdeveloped. It was dry and remote. Its populace was drastically impoverished, deprived, and disadvantaged in every aspect. "We must," said Mayuri Kusump, "help redress their health grievances."[53] In other words, a sense of idealism had permeated the medical profession. Amphon Chindavattana, director of Phanatnikhom hospital in Lopburi who later rose to prominence in the MoPH administration and in its health care reform, commented that serving as the rural practitioner was definitely uncomfortable compared to working with big hospitals in urban cities or in the capital. But running away from such conditions was an easy resolution for someone who had given up. If the rural practitioners were willing to sacrifice their comfort and worked incessantly, their toil would be a great benefit to society.[54]

Despite being imbued with a sense of idealism, the stark reality of the rural conditions was sometimes beyond these young physicians' comprehension. A few cases of death attributed to professional frustration surfaced during the early 1980s.[55] Nevertheless, most illustrative of these incidents was the tragic suicide of Bunthin Samranbamrung. After graduation in 1981, he volunteered to serve in a new community hospital at Maelanoi, far away in the mountainous area of the north. The community was underserved. Electricity would be available only at night, until 10 pm. The public water system was non-existent. Since the area was mountainous, the journey of patients, who were mostly from Thailand's ethnic minorities, to the community hospital was arduous[56] Bunthin arranged a regular mobile service, with a car borrowed from the provincial health headquarters. In one such trip, a car accident injured one of his staff who happened to be the daughter-in-law of the district head who then made threats to Bunthin's life. Bunthin was in a state of nervous collapse and was sent to a hospital in Chiangmai. At the end, Bunthin chose to take his life by jumping from the cliff at Opluang national park on February 24, 1982.[57]

The sacrifice of Bunthin in February 1982 was viewed as the failure of medical schools in coming to terms with the problems in rural health. A few decades later, Komatra Chuengsatiansup, a member of the Society and a graduate of the Chulalongkorn medical school who had been posted to the Chumpuang Hospital, Korat Province, had chosen to pursue his PhD in Anthropology from Harvard in order to better understand the socio-cultural aspects of rural malaise. After having carried out continuous research on Thailand's health system, he published a research manual meant to assist those medical personnel who would engage with primary health care services. For Komatra, this community-based research would offer a new approach in learning about a community's lives as they were, within local socio-cultural and historical contexts.[58] With geo-social mapping, genealogical charts, community organizations, local health systems, local history, community calendars, and life stories, the primary health care service and the community's health conditions could be effectively monitored. For him, a community's health surveillance and primary health care services were not a question of complex medical equipment, but most importantly about an understanding of the community and its socio-cultural context, including an attentiveness to the human condition. Only with these understandings could a health care system that might potentially treat the patients humanely and justly be constructed.[59]

New Hope: A Reform Proposed

Thailand's medical education in the 1960s and 1970s had largely oriented young practitioners toward clinical diagnosis and treatment of individual disease. The Disciplinary Subcommittees' reports for the first national conference on medical education in Thailand, sponsored by the China Medical Board in 1957, highlighted the bias in medical education in the country toward curative care. These curative characteristics were so dominant that Dr. A.E. Brown, a delegate of the WHO office in Saigon, remarked in his speech that though these programs were well-advanced, they did not provide a focus on preventive medicine.[60] But what these young and fresh doctors experienced when they were posted to the rural health centers was rather different from how they had been trained throughout their college years. Suddenly, they became directors of new hospitals and were ill-equipped to cope with administrative matters. In other words, the rural conditions and underdevelopment exposed the stark reality of health care problems that members of the Society were facing.

Politically, this situation had been acknowledged by policy makers and governments since the 1932 revolution that transformed Siam (now known as Thailand) into a constitutional monarchy. Successive policies were implemented to cope with the country's underdevelopment, especially during the height of the Cold War in the 1960s when foreign aid had been pumped into the country. Rural hygiene and the Accelerated Rural Development projects were exemplars of such attempts.

In the opening speech of the 4-week administrative training program for the community hospital's directors at the district level on May 1, 1978, at Savangkhanivas, Samutprakan, Professor Praphon Piyarat (the MoPH deputy minister of the military government and later posted as the WHO's SEARO director of its health human resources during 1979–81) stated clearly that the country's health system was in a state of emergency. If the state of emergency could not be overcome by redressing the inequitable distribution of physicians, the country would eventually succumb to a fate that a few of its neighbors were experiencing, hinting at the communist resurgences in Indochina. The country could only survive when inequities in the access to and availability of public health care were addressed. According to Praphon, the stark disparity in access to health services between Bangkok and the rural areas of Thailand was a kind of social injustice. The country's security and survival depended to a large extent on the well-being of the rural people. For this reason, these hospital directors needed to cooperate with each other to better the people's lives, that is, their well-being, security, and health.[61]

The Rural Doctor Society had searched for a certain kind of reform from the very first year of its founding. Amphon Chindavatthana had once noted with perceptive insight in the Society's journal that all graduated practitioners had been trained mostly in curative medicine. In aspects of prevention, health promotion, sanitation, or self-care, they had only a very general understanding.[62] In tandem with this reform agenda, since 1979, two core members of the Society, that is, Manit Prapansin and Suwit Vibulphonprasert, decided to run for election to the Medical Council of Thailand (MCT)'s board, hoping that they could represent the Society's voice in its policy platform.[63]

Possibly as a result of their advocacy, the MCT established a committee for the continuing medical education of young doctors in September 1980 to which two members of the Society were appointed, namely Manit and Chai Krittayaphichatkul. In the following year, the committee submitted its recommendation that the specialty training program should be controlled more closely in terms of quality and distribution, the addition of regional training institutions, and emphasis on preventive medicine and health rehabilitation. Meanwhile, the committee suggested that the MCT should establish a specific committee for the continuing education of community

Table 4.1 Distribution of Physicians in Thailand, 1977–82

Year	Total	Bangkok and Central Provinces	Northern, Northeast & Southern Provinces	Rural Areas
1977	5,796	3,517	2,279	-
1978	5,899	4,488	1,401	-
1979	~7,386	5,000	2,400	464
1980	6,722	-	-	479
1982	8,644	6,215	2,429	-

Sources: Khanakhammakan phaetthayasapha [Board of the Medical Council of Thailand], "Khosanoenae rueang panha kan phalit phaet lae kan tang khana phaetthayasat mai" [Recommendation on Problems of Physician Production and a Founding of New Faculty of Medicine] (submitted to the Ministerial Council, September 1984), 16–17; "Khrongsang rabop satharanasuk kap kan krachai phaet" [Structure of Public Health System and Physicians' Distribution], *Warasarn chomrom phaetchonnabot*, 3: 2 (1981): 40–43.

hospital physicians in order to improve the training system for general practice appropriate to their environments, to promote on-the-job training at community hospitals, and to reduce the number requested for specialty board training. In other words, a new type of continuing education should be provided to prevent losing these young doctors from rural health work after their training. (In 1981 alone, there were 61 requests of the community hospital doctors for specialty board training; see physicians' distribution during this period in Table 4.1.) Vicharn Panich, a member of the committee and later dean of the Songkhla medical school, also wrote an essay for the journal and suggested that the continuing education should be directed toward the equitable distribution of physicians between the urban and rural areas and toward the integration of curative and preventive medicine, including primary health care, in the rural health service.[64]

In 1981, the Rural Doctor Society argued that as the postgraduate residency programs were not relevant to Thailand's rural needs, the MCT needed to develop short courses for physician administrators serving in the community hospitals.[65] Eventually, the proposal for such a program was submitted to the MCT, drafted by Manit who by then had become a lecturer at Chiangmai medical school.[66] Nevertheless, the MCT committee turned down the proposal, reasoning that the general medicine program should focus on the curative aspect and competency in clinical diagnosis rather than the administrative aspects as suggested. It should be designed for general practitioners, not specific only for physician's administrators in the community hospitals.[67]

Altogether, in advocating for the reform of medical education and the rural health agenda, the Society's journal had routinely explored broader policy-oriented subjects such as primary health care, health economics, pharmaceuticals and consumer protection, the medical specialty board, and tobacco control.[68] Surapong Suebwonglee, the MoPH minister in-charge of health care reform in the early 2000s, also made his political intentions explicit early in his career, saying that he would serve in a community hospital only to carry out his research on public health.[69] Nevertheless, these reform agendas would materialize when core members of the Rural Doctor Society created a shadow strategic college called Sampran Group in 1984, in which a monthly meeting forum was held at Nakhon Pathom to discuss the health care system and policy proposals. A serious study of this policy-oriented think-thank group merits a thorough investigation elsewhere.[70]

Postscript: A Note on Pragmatism

At the beginning, the society clearly had the objective that it would not become involved with politics, apart from focusing on rural public health care problems and supporting medical practitioners working in the rural health care centers and community hospitals. Nevertheless, within a year the non-association with politics was changed to "promote the [social] status of rural medical practitioners."[71]

A recent publication, in which one among its three authors was a former member of the society, that is, Komatra Chuengsatiansup, contended that the society's approach was, and still is, John Dewey's pragmatic instrumentalism and Paul Farmer's pragmatic solidarity.[72] Taking this stance, in their perspective, the society could push forward with arduous tasks, either during authoritarian or democratic governments, especially in articulating regulations or policies that were in stark conflict to the capitalist interests during authoritarian regimes established by military coups. From their perspective, the pragmatic position would be understandably resisted by those who had power and interests in the "old structure" that struggled to retain its dominant status and by those "dogmatic idealists" who guard their principles like a sacred canon and refuse to compromise them. Pragmatism is not a bad thing in itself, they argue, especially in dealing with illness that is intimately related to matters of life and death. A dogmatic principle without elasticity, they reason, could be a hindrance in mobilizing for an important issue. Pragmatism could be acceptable, therefore, as long as their movement's objective was directed, not to themselves, but to the benefit of those who are less well-off.[73]

It is notable that the "old structure," in their perspective, did actually mean the socio-political structure that was a blend of modern bureaucracy and liberal capitalism that has been emerging since the introduction of constitutional monarchy in 1932.[74] Ironically, the Rural Doctor Society, as a "progressive structure," always joined ranks with the structure put in place by the military juntas, right-wing bureaucrats and the network monarchy.[75] Apparently, as the COVID-19 pandemic is claiming people's lives and the vaccine administration of the military government is undeniably in a state of failure, leaders of the Rural Doctor Society chose to remain silent or make a rather gentle remark about the situation, in contrast to the loud noise they had made during the prior elected government.

The current COVID-19 crisis in Thailand reveals that despite the lack of political leadership on the part of Thai government, the country's health system has been able to effectively manage the pandemic. Unlike Hong Kong or Taiwan, the Thai government adopted an Economy First approach and was reluctant to seal its borders to tourists, especially those from China, for fear of losing foreign exchange. In January 2020, Anutin Chanvirakul, the Thai Minister of Health, downplayed the COVID-19 pandemic, saying that it was akin to the old common cold.[76] The next month, the Minister backpedaled and admitted the gravity of the situation.[77] To stem the spread of the virus, the government imposed the first of a series of lockdowns between March 26 and April 30, 2020.

Caught between a rock and a hard place without any kind of social security, Bangkok's migrant workers fled to their hometowns, crowding bus terminals and stoking fears of spreading COVID-19 to the hinterland. With the cancelation of Thai New Year festivities in April 2020, families of migrant workers were unable to share food on the table. To mitigate the fallout of the crisis, the government announced in April 2020, the 5000-baht scheme (US$160) cash handout for informal workers.[78] Several complications ensued such as erroneous screening and fraudulent claims. The government's relief measures for small-scale business were limited to extending the tax deadline. And the meager relief measures could be attributed to the government's unwillingness to incur public debts.

Despite stopgap measures of the government to stem the tide of COVID-19, the health system of Thailand has shown considerable resilience in the wake of the pandemic. In the Global Health Security Index, the country occupies sixth position.[79] The resilience of Thailand's health system could be attributed to the country's National Health Development Plan (1960–75). In response to this long-term plan, the government established a network of district hospitals, beginning in 1977. Village Health Volunteers or Community Health Workers (CHW)—introduced in 1977 as a part of the government's plan to expand healthcare to rural areas, in response to the demands from the Rural Doctor Society— were in the forefront of the fight against COVID-19. During the exodus of migrant workers to rural areas, the CHW played a pivotal role in educating workers' families about COVID-19. With rudimentary training in primary health, many CHWs are diagnosed COVID-19 in remote areas. In this pandemic emergency, the evolution of the Rural Doctor Society during the 1970s and the 1980s is illustrative of the transitional period in Thailand's health care reform when first-class physicians were posted to remote rural areas. At that particular moment, the rural doctors and the community health workers encountered one another and joined forces, which is another story waiting to be told.

Acknowledgments

In preparing this essay, I have greatly benefited from comments, suggestions, and help of whom I owe enormous gratitude, especially

Vivek Neelakantan, Craig J. Reynolds, Trais Pearson, Chalong Soontravanich, Sikha Songkumchum, Krijakara Kokpuak, Thobodi Buakamsri, Chatchai Muksong, Tapanik Tisase, Siwakorn Ratchompoo, Nathatai Manadee, and anonymous reviewers.

Notes

1 See Sombat Chantornvong, "To Address the Dust of the Dust Under the Soles of the Royal Feet: A Reflection on the Political Dimension of the Thai Court Language," *Asian Review* 6 (1992): 144–63.

2 See Davisakd Puaksom, "Of Germs, Public Hygiene, and the Healthy Body: The Making of the Medicalizing State in Thailand," *Journal of Asian Studies* 66, no. 2 (May 2007): 311–44.

3 See Duncan McCargo and Ukrist Pathmanand, *The Thaksinization of Thailand* (Copenhagen: NIAS Press, 2004); Duncan McCargo, *Fighting for Virtue: Justice and Politics in Thailand* (Ithaca: Cornell University Press, 2020); *Coup, King, Crisis: A Critical Interregnum in Thailand*, Pavin Chachavalpongpun edited (New Haven: Yale Southeast Asia Studies, 2021).

4 See Xiaoping Fang, *Barefoot Doctors and Western Medicine in China* (Rochester: University of Rochester Press, 2012); Liping Bu, "The Patriotic Health Movement and China's Socialist Reconstruction: Fighting Disease and Transforming Society, 1950–80," in *Public Health and National Reconstructions in Post-War Asia: International Influences, Local Transformations*, Liping Bu and Ka-che Yip edited (London and New York: Routledge, 2014), 34–51; and Xun Zhou, *The People's Health: Health Intervention and Delivery in Mao's China, 1949–1983* (Montreal & Kingston: McGill-Queen's University Press, 2020).

5 Vivek Neelakantan, *Science, Public Health, and Nation-Building in Soekarno-Era Indonesia* (Newcastle: Cambridge Scholars Publishing, 2017), 67–91; see also Margaret Jones, *Striving for Equity: Healthcare in Sri Lanka from Independence to the Millennium, 1948–2000* (Hyderabad: Orient BlackSwan, 2020).

6 Teresa S. Encarnacion Tadem, "The Role of Non-governmental Organizations in the Field of Health in Modern Southeast Asia: The Philippine Experience," in *Histories of Health in Southeast Asia: Perspectives on the Long Twentieth Century*, Tim Harper and Sunil S. Amrith edited (Bloomington and Indianapolis: Indiana University Press, 2014), 222–25.

7 For example, Viroj Tangcharoensathien, Woranan Witthayapipopsakul, Warisa Panichkriangkrai, Walaiporn Patcharanarumol, and Anne Mills, "Health Systems Development in Thailand: A Solid Platform for Successful Implementation of Universal Health Coverage," *The Lancet* (January 31, 2018): 1–18; Woranan Witthayapipopsakul, Anond Kulthanmanusorn, Vuthiphan Vongmongkol, Shaheda Viriyathorn, Yaowaluk Wanwong, and Viroj Tangcharoensathien, "Achieving the Targets for Universal Health Coverage: How Is Thailand Monitoring Progress?" *WHO South-East Asia Journal of Public Health* 8, no.1 (April 2019): 10–17.

8 Illan Nam, *Democratizing Health Care: Welfare State Building in Korea and Thailand* (New York: Palgrave, 2015), 169–204; Joseph Harris, *Achieving Access: Professional Movements and the Politics of Universal Health Care* (Ithaca and London: Cormell University Press, 2017), 35–62 and chapter 5. Apparently, this inclination also includes two dissertations in Thai, that is, Chettha Sapyen, "Kan sueksa khabuankan phaetchonnabot nai krabuankan kamnot nayobai rabop sukhapap: khabuankan patirup phachasangkhom

songphon to prachathippatai baep mi suanruam nai phrathet thai" [A Study of Rural Doctor Movement in the Policy Process of Health System Policy: The Movement of Civil Society and Its Contribution Toward Participatory Democracy in Thailand] (PhD dissertation, Politics, Chulalongkorn University, 2013) and Nattarute Vongtangswad, "Phonlawat krap khwam khit lae kan khluanwai khong khabuan kan phaetchonnabot: khwam khatyaeng lae kan plianphan thang kanmuang" [The Dynamics of Framing and Mobilization of the Rural Doctor Movement: Conflicts and Political Transformation] (PhD dissertation, Politics, Chulalongkorn University, 2017).

9   Nam, *Democratizing Health Care*, 174.

10   For the international context refer Victor W. Sidel, "The Barefoot Doctors of the People's Republic of China," *New England Journal of Medicine* 286, no. 24 (1972): 1292–300; Victor W. Sidel and Ruth Sidel, "The Health Care Delivery System of the People's Republic of China," in *Health by the People*, Kenneth W. Newell edited (Geneva: World Health Organization, 1975), 1–12; Socrates Litsios, "The Long and Difficult Road to Alma-Ata: A Personal Reflection," *International Journal of Health Service* 32, no. 4 (2002): 709–32; Anne-Emanuelle Birn and Nikolai Krementsov, "'Socialising' Primary Care? The Soviet Union, WHO and the 1978 Alma-Ata Conference," *BMJ Global Health* 3 (2018): e000992, DOI:10.1136/bmjgh-2018-0009. For a fine-grained analysis of the Barefoot Doctor Model refer Peter Worsley, "Non-Western Medical System," *Annual Review of Anthropology* 11, no. 2 (1982): 315–48; See also Fang, *Barefoot Doctors and Western Medicine in China*, 2 and 204.

11   Harris, "A Right to Health?," 45–83.

12   See Davisakd Puaksom, "A Promise of Desire: On the Politics of Health Care and Moral Discourse in Thailand, 1950–2010," in *Public Health and National Reconstructions in Post-War Asia*, Liping Bu and Ka-che Yip edited (London and New York: Routledge, 2014), 176–85.

13   See Thak Chaloemtiarana, *Thailand: The Politics of Despotic Paternalism* (Ithaca, New York: Cornell Southeast Asian Program, 2007), 81–110.

14   Sulak Sivaraksa, *Ha pi chak parithat khong S. Sivaraksa* [Five Years from Social Science Review of Sulak Sivaraksa] (Bangkok: Sueksitsayam Press, 1969); Prajak Kongkirati, *Laelaew khwam khluanwai ko prakot: kanmuang vatthanatham khong naksueksa lae panyachon khon 14 tula* [As the Movement Emerges: Cultural Politics of Students and Intellectuals Before 14 October 1973] (Bangkok: Thammasat University Press, 2005).

15   Harris, "A Right to Health?" 61.

16   See similar attempts of the Indonesian government in regulating an inequitable distribution of physicians in Neelakantan, *Science, Public Health, and Nation-Building in Soekarno-Era Indonesia*, 78–80; Vivek Neelakantan, "The Expansion and Transformation of Medical Education in Indonesia during the 1950s in Jakarta and Surabaya," in *Translating the Bodies: Medical Educating in Southeast Asia*, Hans Pols, C. Michele Thompson and John Harley Warner edited (Singapore: NUS Press, 2017), 173–93. For the proposal to decentralizing health care to rural areas in the Philippine, see Vivek Neelakantan, "'No Nation Can Go Forward When It is Crippled by Disease': Philippine Science and the Cold War, 1946–65," *Southeast Asian Studies* 10, no.1 (2021): 53–87.

17   "Kan chatsan phaet" [Medical Practitioners Distribution], *Warasan chomrom phaetchonnabot*, 3: 4 (1981): 20–22; "Chatakam phaet rapthun run 10" [Fate of Grant Recipient Practitioners Cohort No.10], *Warasan chomrom phaetchonnabot* 3, no. 4 (1981): 23–28; "Kwamkhithen khong phaet rapthun runthi 1" [Opinion of a First Cohort of Grant Recipient Practitioners], *Warasan chomrom phaetchonnabot* 3, no. 4 (1981): 9–10.

18 Suwit Wibulpolprasert edited, *25 pi khabuankan phaetchonnabot kap phaendin thai* [25 Years of the Rural Doctor Movement in Thailand] (Bangkok: WHO, 2003), 226–27.

19 Scott Bamber, "The Thai Medical Profession and Political Activism," in *Political Change in Thailand: Democracy and Participation*, in Kevin Hewison edited (London and New York: Routledge, 1997), 235–36; see also Paul T. Cohen, "Public Health in Thailand: Changing Medical Paradigms and Disease Patterns in Political and Economic Context," 106–21, in *Public Health in Asia and the Pacific: Historical and Comparative Perspectives*, Milton J. Lewis and Kerrie L. MacPherson edited (London: Routledge, 2007), 110–13.

20 See Kanokrat Lertchoosakul, *The Rise of the Octobrists in Contemporary Thailand: Power and Conflict among Former Left-Wing Student Activists in Thai Politics* (New Haven: Yale University Southeast Asia Studies, 2016), chapter 2.

21 See Tyrell Haberkorn, *Revolution Interrupted: Farmers, Students, Law, and Violence in Northern Thailand* (Madison: University of Wisconsin Press, 2011).

22 Suwit, *25 pi khabuankan phaetchonnabot*, 1–10; Racha Putchong, Noppanat Anuphongphat, and Komatra Chuengsatirasap, *Phaetchonnabot: Thammaphiban kap kanmuang sukkhaphap* [The Rural Doctors: Good Governance and Health Politics] (Nonthaburi: Health System Research Institute, 2013), 48.

23 Suwit, *25 pi khabuankan phaetchonnabot*, 10–11. A parallel process in Indonesia could be seen during the 1970s. See, for example, Januar Achmad, *Hollow Development: The Politics of Health in Soeharto's Indonesia* (Canberra: The Australian National University, 1999), chapter 5.

24 Benedict Anderson, "Withdrawal Symptoms: Social and Cultural Aspects of the October 6 Coup," *Bulletin of Concerned Asian Scholars* 9, no.3 (1977): 13–30; Thongchai Winichakul, *Moments of Silence: The Unforgetting of the October 6, 1976, Massacre in Bangkok* (Honolulu: University of Hawaii Press, 2020), chapter 2.

25 For example, see Puttapon Mongkolworawan, "Phabuankan communist nai khet phuphan, pho.so.2504–2525" [The Communist Movement in Phuphan Area, 1961–1982] (MA thesis, Chulalongkorn University, 2005); Ian G. Baird, "The Hmong and the Communist Party of Thailand: A Transnational, Transcultural and Gender-Relations-Transforming Experience," *TRaNS: Trans-Regional and -National Studies of Southeast Asia* 9, no. 2 (2021): 1–18.

26 Suwit, *25 pi khabuankan phaetchonnabot*, 227–28; for Vichai's account of his personal experience, see Vichai Chokevivat, *Liawlang laena: 60 pi moh Vichai Chokevivat* [Reflecting Backward, Eying Forward: 60 Years of Dr Vichai Chokevivat] (Bangkok: Komol Khimthong Foundation, 2007), 10–19.

27 Haberkorn, *Revolution Interrupted*, 105–28; Bamber, "The Thai Medical Profession and Political Activism," 237.

28 While the first three have become prominent politicians, the last one was a professor of medicine at Songkhla medical school.

29 Suwit, *25 pi khabuankan phaetchonnabot*, 228–29.

30 Ibid., 11–12.

31 See minute of their first general meeting and name-list of the participants in *Warasan chomrom phaetchonnabot* 1, no. 1 (June 1978), 13–16. Other active members that did not appear in the name-list, from Suwit's recollection, were Prasop Phonphai, Khom Pongkhan, Chalo Guptavindhu, Luecha Vanarat, Chuchai Supavong, Amphon Chindavattana, Sanguan Nittayaramphong, and Somsak Chunharas. See Suwit, *25 pi khabuankan phaetchonnabot*, 5. The denomination of this group were sometime printed in English in their journal as "The Rural Doctor Association." Nevertheless, "The Rural Doctor

Society" would be called here as it was already well-known. Generally, the federation was designated for a political organ of the leftist or left-leaning movement, for example the Federation of Thailand's Peasants and Farmers, the name change here was undoubtedly a political strategy to distancing the society from the revolutionary fervour and avoiding suppression. Nevertheless, the political stance of the society was rather ambiguous; and few active members of the society were later disclosed as key figures or alliances of the CPT underground elements.

32 See Randall M. Packard, *A History of Global Health: Interventions into the Lives of Other Peoples* (Baltimore: Johns Hopkins University Press, 2016).

33 Davisakd, "A Promise of Desire," 176–80; see also Thak, *Thailand*, 147–79.

34 Ibid., 181–83.

35 Fang, *Barefoot Doctors and Western Medicine in China*, 28–33; Zhou, *The People's Health*, 178–256.

36 Pricha Disawat, "Kan satharanasukmunthan nai prathetthat" [The Primiary Health Care in Thailand] (Office of the Primary Health Care Commission, 1980); Tawithong Hongwiwat, "Khrongkan satharanasukmunthan" [The Primary Health Care Project] (A Study for the Rural Development, Office of the National Commission for the Economic and Social Development, 1981), 4–5. On state's intervention of traditional midwife, see Claudia Merli, *Bodily Practices and Medical Identities in Southern Thailand* (Uppsala: Acta Universitatis Upsaliensis, Uppsala Studies in Cultural Anthropology, 2008) and "Muslim midwives between traditions and modernities: Being and becoming a *bidan kampung* in Satun province, Southern Thailand," *Moussons* 15 (2010): 121–35.

37 Tawithong Hongwiwat, Supot Denduang, and Netnapha Khumthong, "Rongphayaban amphoe nai prathetthai: kan sueksa choeng nayobai" [Community Hospital in Thailand: A Policy Study] (Public Health Policy Paper, Center of Public Health Policy, Mahidol University, 1982), 4–5.

38 See Marcos Cueto, "The Origins of Primary Health Care and Selective Primary Health Care," *American Journal of Public Health* 94, no. 11 (November 2004): 1864–74; WHO and United Nations Children's Fund, *Primary Health Care* (Geneva and New York: International Conference on Primary Health Care, Alma-Ata, USSR, 6–12 September 1978); Packard, *A History of Global Health*, part IV.

39 In volume 7, edited by Viravat Phankrut, the journal printed its name in English as *The Rural Doctor Association Bulletin*. But to avoid confusion with another monthly publication of the Society, the *Warasan* would be translated here as the Society's journal. Later in 1979, the Society also published another periodical called *Chulasan chomrom phaetchonnabot* [Bulletin of the Rural Doctor Society] that focused mainly on the Society's operations and matters directly related to its members.

40 "Khwampenma khong chomrom phaetchonnabot" [Background of the Rural Doctor Society], *Warasan chomrom phaetchonnabot* 1, no. 1 (June 1978), 1.

41 "Rabiap chomrom phaetchonnabot" [Regulations of the Rural Doctor Society], *Warasan chomrom phaetchonnabot* 1, no. 1 (June 1978), 3. For a comparative perspective on the physicians' community involvement in Indonesian and Philippine's rural health development, see Achmad, *Hollow Development*, 89–98; and Neelakantan, "No Nation Can Go Forward When It Is Crippled by Disease," 78–81.

42 "Sarayaniyakorn Thalaeng" [Editorial Foreword], *Warasan chomrom phaetchonnabot* 1, no. 1 (June 1978), 2.

43 This romantic phrase appeared in Amphon Chindavattana, "Choen ruamsang thangsaimai" [Let Us Build a New Road], *Warasan chomrom phaetchonnabot* 2, no. 1 (June–August 1979): 3–6. There was a well known story of a young

doctor, Apichet Naklekha, who was dispatched to work in the remote rural area, at Prao hospital, Chiang Mai. A collection of letters and writings relating his experience there was published and widely read among leftists and activists in the 1970s. Notably, Apichet's life and works greatly inspired later generations of young physicians to work for the rural health improvement. In 1979, just a few years after the Rural Doctor Society was organized, Apichet's story was also adapted to the silver screen, directed by Charin Thongsin. See Apichet Naklekha, *Moh mueang proa* [A Doctor at Prao City] (Bangkok: Khonnum, 1976).

44 "Rongphayaban huasai nakhonsrithammarat" [Huasai Hospital, Nakhon Sri Thammarat], *Warasan chomrom phaetchonnabot* 1, no. 2 (September 1978): 30–32.

45 "Chiwit khong phaetying" [Female Doctor's Life], *Warasan chomrom phaetchonnabot* 1, no. 4 (March 1979): 20–23.

46 Amphon Chindavattana, "Prasopkan khong mohbannok khonnueng" [Experience of a Rural Doctor], *Warasan chomrom phaetchonnabot* 2, no. 2 (December 1979–February 1980): 30–33.

47 "Naiphaet Viput Puncharoen" [Doctor Viput Puncharoen], *Warasan chomrom phaetchonnabot* 1, no. 4 (March 1979): 29–32.

48 "Samphat naiphaet Chai Kritiyapichatkul" [Interview of Doctor Chai Kritiyapichatkul], *Chulasan chomrom phaetchonnabot* 4, no. 8 (December 1982): 9–13.

49 Amphon Chindavattana, "Khwan" [Spirit], *Warasan chomrom phaetchonnabot* 1, no. 4 (March 1979): 18–19; Vivat Rojanaphithayakorn, "Khwan krachoeng" [Spirited Away], 2, no. 2 (December 1979–February 1980): 18–20. On discussion of the "khwan," see Trais Pearson, *Sovereign Necropolis: The Politics of Death in Semi-Colonial Siam* (Ithaka and London: Cornell University Press, 2020), 169–73.

50 "Chotmai" [A Letter], *Warasan chomrom phaetchonnabot* 3, no. 4 (1981): 51–52.

51 See Fred W. Riggs, *Thailand: The Modernization of a Bureaucratic Polity* (Honolulu: East-West Center Press, 1966); Ralph Thaxton, "Modernization and Counter-Revolution in Thailand," *Bulletin of Concerned Asian Scholars* 5, no. 4 (1973): 28–40.

52 Vichai Chokevivat, "Khokhit chak phappayon" [A Thought from Cinema], *Chulasan chomrom phaetchonnabot* 4, no. 10 (1983): 25–31, cf.29.

53 "Chiwit khong phaetying," 23.

54 Amphon, "Choen ruamsang thangsaimai," 4–5. Definitely, a sense of idealism permeating the medical profession was hardly new; see a similar rhetoric of doctors serving in Indonesian rural areas in Neelakantan, *Science, Public Health, and Nation-Building in Soekarno-Era Indonesia*, 77–78.

55 See, for example, "Khwamtai khong Nanthaphon: Tairomyem chingrue?" [A Death of Doctor Nanthaphon: Is the South Really Peaceful?], *Chulasan chomrom phaetchonnabot* 4, no. 1 (1982).

56 For a glimpse of highland ethnic studies in Thailand, see Kwanchewan Buadaeng, "The Rise and Fall of the Tribal Research Institute (TRI): 'Hill Tribe' Policy and Studies in Thailand," *Southeast Asian Studies* 44, no. 3 (December 2006): 359–84.

57 Phaetphuthorn [Rural Doctor], "Siangtakone khong moh Bunthin" [The Outcry of Doctor Bunthin], *Chulasan chomrom phaetchonnabot* 4, no. 1 (1982).

58 Komatra Chuengsatiansup, *Vithi chumchon* [Community's Path], first published in 2002, 10th edition (Nonthaburi: Society and Health Institute, 2012), preface.

59 Ibid., 13.

60 See "Ruam rai-ngan kanprachum kan op-romsueksa phaetthayasat khong thai krang raek" [Proceeding Reports of First Conference on Thailand's Medical Education], organized by University of Medicine, Ministry of Public Health, Bangsaen, Chonburi Province, 25–30 November 1957; see Brown's remark in A. E. Brown, "Kham prasai" [Speech], in "Ruam rai-ngan kanprachum kan op-romsueksa phaetthayasat khong thai krang raek," 194–96. See also the medical education reform in the 1950s Indonesia in Neelakantan, "The Expansion and Transformation of Medical Education in Indonesia During the 1950s in Jakarta and Surabaya," 173–93.

61 "Khamklaw poet kan-oprom danborihan" [Opening Address for the Administrative Training], *Warasan chomrom phaetchonnabot* 1, no. 2 (September 1978), 20–21. For a brief biography of Praphon, see *Anusorn ngan phrarat-chathanploengsop sattrachan naiphaet praphon piyarat* [A Cremation Volume of Professor Praphon Piyarat] (Wat Makuttriyaram, Bangkok, 7 March 1998).

62 Amphon, "Choen ruamsang thangsaimai," 6.

63 Both were later voted as elected members of the MCT's board in 1982 in which Suwit had become its youngest member since the MCT's board was founded in 1968. Thereafter, other members of the Society joined the league, for instances, Vichai Chokevivat and Chuchai Supavongs. During 1986–92, the Society was very active in the MCT in which its member served as the secretariat of the MCT board during 1987–95. See Suwit Vibulpolprasert, *Do It Right and Fear No Man* (Bangkok: IHPP and HITAP, 2013), 82.

64 Vicharn Panich, "Khosanoenae naikan chatkansueksa phaet tonueang phoe hai koet 'Health for All by the Year 2000'" [A Recommendation for the Continuing Education of Physicians in Order to Achieve 'Health for All by the Year 2000'], *Warasan chomrom phaetchonnabot* 3, no. 2 (1981): 25–26.

65 See Somjit Prueksaritanond and Prasong Tuchinda, "General Practice Residency Training Program in Thailand: Past, Present, and Future," *Journal of Medical Association* 84 (2001): 1153–55; See also Amphon Chindavattana, "Phaet ropo-or kap 'board'," *Warasan chomrom phaetchonnabot* 3, no. 2 (1981): 13–14; "Phaet ropo-or pairienboard kanmak" [Massive Rural Hospital's Doctors Had Continued Their Specialty Training], *Warasan chomrom phaetchonnabot* 3, no. 2 (1981): 32–33.

66 "Khosanoe khong chomrom phaetchonnabot hai phaetsapha chat-oprom phaetvetchapatipat tuapai samrap phaet ropo-or" [Rural Doctor Society's Proposal to the Medical Council to Have a Training Program on General Practitioners for the Rural Hospital's Doctors], *Chulasan chomrom phaetchonnabot* 3, no. 2 (1981): 34–39.

67 "Nathi lae botbat khong phaetthayasapha nai kan sueksatonueang khong phaet" [Functions and Roles of the Medical Council of Thailand for the Continuing Medical Education], *Warasan chomrom phaetchonnabot* 3, no. 2 (1981): 27–31. For a comparison, with Indonesia, see Neelakantan, "The Expansion and Transformation of Medical Education in Indonesian during the 1950s in Jakarta and Surabaya," 180–82.

68 See articles and commentaries on the primary health care in *Warasan chomrom phaetchonnabot* 2, no. 3 (1982); on the health care economics in *Warasan chomrom phaetchonnabot* 6, no.3 (1986); on pharmaceuticals in *Warasan chomrom phaetchonnabot* 8, no. 2 (1988); on specialty board in *Warasan chomrom phaetchonnabot* 3, no. 2 (1981); and on tobacco control in *Warasan chomrom phaetchonnabot* 7, no. 3 (1987) and *Chulasan chomrom phaetchonnabot* 12, no. 3 (1989).

69 "Khao chomrom" [Society's News], *Chulasan chomrom phaetchonnabot* 4, no. 10 (1983): 21–23, cf.22.

70 Suwit, *25 pi khabuankan phaetchonnabot*, 56–70.
71 *Warasan chomrom phaetchonnabot* [Journal of the Society of the Rural Doctors], 1, no. 4 (1979); cited in Suwit, *25 pi khabuankan phaetchonnabot*, 12.
72 Racha, Noppanat and Komatra, *Phaetchonnabot*, 9–10. See also John Dewey, *The Quest for Certainty: A Study of the Revelation of Knowledge and Action* (New York: Minton, Balch & Company, 1929); and Paul Farmer, *Pathologies of Power: Health, Human Rights, and the New War on the Poor* (Los Angeles: University of California Press, 2004).
73 Ibid., 181–84.
74 See Kobkua Suwannathat-Pian, *Thailand's Durable Premier: Phibun through Three Decades, 1932–1957* (London: Oxford University Press, 1995); Puli Fuwongcharoen, "'Long Live Ratthathammanūn!': Constitution Worship in Revolutionary Siam," *Modern Asian Studies* 52, no. 2 (2018): 609–44.
75 See Duncan McCargo, "Network Monarchy and Legitimacy Crises in Thailand," *The Pacific Review* 18, no. 4 (2005): 499–519; Lotte Isager and Soren Ivarsson, *Saying the Unsayable: Monarchy and Democracy in Thailand* (Copenhagen: NIAS, 2010).
76 Anonymous, "COVID-19 Response in Thailand," *CSEAS Newsletter* 78 (June 8, 2020), https://covid-19chronicles.cseas.kyoto-u.ac.jp/post-044-html/.
77 Ibid.
78 Ibid.
79 Alwin Issac, R.V. Radhakrishnan, V.R. Vijay, S. Stephen, N. Krishnan, J. Jacob, S. Jose, S.M. Azhar, and A.S. Nair, "An Examination of Thailand's Health Care System and Strategies During the Management of the COVID-19 Pandemic, *Journal of Global Health* 11 (2021): 03002. DOI: https://doi.org/10.7189%2Fjogh.11.03002.

5   Civic Space in the Time of COVID-19

The Case of Maritime Southeast Asia

Khoo Ying Hooi

Introduction

On March 11, 2020, the World Health Organization declared COVID-19 a pandemic since it burst into headlines in Wuhan, China in December 2019. Between March 2020 and March 2021, the virus infected over 118 million people globally and killed 2.6 million.[1] The associated lockdowns have devastated economies and upended political orders or have solidified them. COVID-19 has impacted Southeast Asia in many ways. First, the region witnessed an economic recession not witnessed since the Asian financial crisis of 1998. Every economy of the region, excluding Vietnam, contracted due to the COVID-19-induced recession. Second, statistics fail to communicate personal hardships that resulted from COVID-19 lockdowns. Third, the World Bank has estimated that the number of poor people in Southeast Asia is set to rise for the first time in 20 years due to a combination of job losses and school closures that in turn, would lead to erosion of human capital. The pandemic has underscored the brute fact of Southeast Asia's close proximity and entwinement with rising China whose own economic recovery is important in the region's attempt to pull itself out of pandemic-induced recession. Southeast Asian nations are trying to balance their national anxiety stemming from Beijing's growing belligerence on the one hand, with the desire to benefit from economic partnership with their giant neighbor, on the other.

Politically, the pandemic has accelerated the reactionary wave of the past decade by giving opportunity to autocratic leaders such as Rodrigo Duterte of the Philippines to equip themselves with emergency powers and impose restrictions on political opponents. The trend has been opposed by the emergence of an anti-authoritarian protest movement, setting the stage for political crises in many Southeast Asian countries.[2]

Since 2020, various political analysts have shown how a global health crisis such as the ongoing COVID-19 pandemic has complicated the discourse on democracy and human rights.[3] This chapter looks at the situation in Southeast Asia. The ASEAN (Association of Southeast Asian Nations)—a regional grouping comprising Myanmar, Thailand, Vietnam, Cambodia,

DOI: 10.4324/9781003332060-6

Laos, Malaysia, Indonesia, Singapore, Brunei, and the Philippines, established in 1967—has recognized the importance of preventing the spread of disease through the adaptation of the International Health Regulations (IHR) introduced by the WHO in 2005. Despite vastly different political systems and varying health capacities, ASEAN nations accepted the internalization of IHR. The convergence of views of individual member states of the region and the WHO led to the introduction of APSED (Asia Pacific Strategy for Emerging Infectious Diseases) in 2005. The APSED set minimum benchmarks for ASEAN members for reporting infectious outbreaks.[4] However, the acceptance of IHR contradicted the behavior from the same member states that opposed imposition of international norms, in other areas such as recognition of civil and political rights and refugee status recognition.[5]

The lack of formal legislative and funding mechanisms and dependence on elite political relationships to progress reforms make ASEAN a weak political body to promote change.[6] The "ASEAN Way" has caused decision-making processes to be slow and politicized. The primacy of national sovereignty, the prevalence of national interests over collective good, and the culture of rule by consensus have been the main obstacles to collective action by member states.

Focusing on the Southeast Asia region, however, this chapter omits mainland Southeast Asia. It will specifically focus on maritime Southeast Asia—also ASEAN member states—namely, Brunei, Indonesia, Malaysia, the Philippines, and Singapore. Before the analysis is being made, it is essential to understand the context of the five selected countries. Among ASEAN states, Indonesia is the most populous, whereas Brunei and Singapore are among the least. Between the 1980s and the early 2000s, Southeast Asia was the hub of a global wave of democratization. For instance, the Philippines underwent political fermentation in 1986—the People Power Revolution (EDSA)—that resulted in the non-violent overthrow of the two-decade-long Marcos dictatorship. In a similar vein, Indonesia underwent democratization in 1998 following the overthrow of the Suharto *Orde Baru* (New Order) regime (1967–98). The Asian financial crisis (1997) was the proximate cause that accounted for President Suharto's downfall and questioned the developmentalist narrative of the *Orde Baru*.[7] At the same time, the financial crisis undermined the credibility of Malaysia's modernity trope that was focused on maintaining economic growth and ethnic harmony. The ouster of the then Malaysian Deputy Prime Minister Anwar Ibrahim set the stage for the *Reformasi* (Political Reform) movement, an organized mass protest movement that embraced a range of socio-political actors that included non-governmental organizations, grassroots movements, and political parties. However, since the late 2000s, the region has regressed politically, part of a global wave of democratic backsliding that seems to be gathering pace.[8]

The political system in each of the five countries studied is diverse with a mixture of democratic and authoritarian elements. Moreover, their economic levels are unequal. The categorization of countries into different groups is divided across different indexes. The five countries can be divided into two categories. The first category is inclusive of developed countries, namely Brunei and Singapore. Both Brunei and Singapore are among the wealthiest countries based on the World Bank 2020 GDP per capita data. Yet their emergency measures are intensifying ongoing processes of democratic backsliding and have arguably left negative repercussions on the inclusiveness of ASEAN, which is expected to be people-oriented.[9]

Southeast Asian nations do not have a good record on democracy and human rights. The COVID-19 crisis has pushed the five countries discussed in the chapter into different variations of a lockdown. In the chapter, I contend that lockdowns afford regimes with authoritarian tendencies the opportunity to suppress political dissents further and consolidate their power.[10] This raises concerns particularly among the civil society actors working on human rights and democracy that "a state of emergency" enforced by political leaders in maritime Southeast Asia might become a permanent fixture that could erode the nascent democratic institutions further, particularly in the case of Indonesia, Malaysia, and the Philippines. How leaders and their citizens interact during the coronavirus crisis could also provide some clues to the future exercise of political power. The approaches adopted by the five countries also raise the question of the weaponization of COVID-19. Recognizing these issues, this chapter examines how pandemic restrictions have impacted the civic space of Brunei, Indonesia, Malaysia, the Philippines, and Singapore, respectively. In doing so, this chapter gathers data from the official documents of the five countries on their COVID-19 measures. The data of the democracy index from the Economist Intelligence Unit (EIU) and the civic space from the CIVICUS Monitor are also employed in this chapter.

The Discourse on Securitization

In the literature of International Relations (IR), especially in security studies, securitization is often used to denote how a state securitizes an issue to block a threat. In many ways, securitization is also employed as a concept and a theory within IR literature. With the arrival of the COVID-19—which has impacted the whole region and disrupted how the international system functions—there has been a burgeoning scholarship that seeks to link both securitization and COVID-19 and investigate the ways in which a state securitizes the pandemic to contain its spread and to protect life.[11] However, securitization of the pandemic can lead to an erosion of civil and political rights.

The concept of securitization has evolved in response to significant world events. In the late 1970s, Michel Foucault predicted that the international community would increasingly live in a "society of security."[12] For Foucault, modern society was moving in a direction increasingly typified by prevailing discourses of securitization, which underpinned a governmentalized world of regulated political, economic, and social subjectivity.[13] The securitization theory was developed by Copenhagen School scholars such as Barry Buzan, Ole Wæver, and Jaap de Wilde, who are mainly concerned with respect to how security is socially constructed in international politics and the extent to which political actors view and construct specific issues as security threats.[14] For instance, Buzan, Waever and de Wilde define securitization as a speech act that fulfils three rhetorical criteria.[15] It is a discursive process through which an actor claims that a referent object is existentially threatened, demands the right to take extraordinary countermeasures to deal with the threat, and convinces an audience that rule-breaking behavior to counter the threat is justified. The securitization theory emphasizes the role of the speech act in framing an issue as an existential threat to a referent's survival and well-being.[16]

Securitization, however, is not only limited to speech acts but also includes securitizing practices such as those employed by authoritarian regimes.[17] If accepted by the audience, the securitization process allows the state to suspend typical political methods and use emergency measures in response to the crisis. In this sense, security can be seen as a place of negotiation between securitizing actors and the audience. The audience will accept securitization based on a series of four "facilitating conditions": (a) concerns of security; (b) the social capital of the securitizing actors; (c) conditions related to threat; and (d) conditions related to the audience.[18]

Since 1992, IR scholars have linked health issues to the securitization theory.[19] Over the past 30 years, global diseases such as HIV/AIDS, SARS, Ebola, or Zika were presented as threats and carefully securitized by different countries at the international level.[20] COVID-19 was hardly different. Governments and scientists in the health crisis arrogated themselves to the role of securitizing actors to showcase how COVID-19 could be a threat to people's lives, the state, health services, and society such that they could justify draconian measures including adherence to lockdowns, or deploy the military on the streets to enforce pandemic-related protocols.[21] Indonesian IR expert Tangguh Chairil contends that there are benefits of securitizing health issues: on the security side, public health experts bring valuable tools and expertise to a few new problems, while on the health side, public health securitization raises its political profile leading to the prospect of more significant resources devoted to urgent health needs.[22]

Securitization is most often linked with the act of militarization in terms of the emergency methods used by the state to respond to an existential threat.[23] Militarization is defined as the accumulation of capacity for organized violence and measures the extent of use of military structures and procedures in a state's decision-making process.[24] In the pandemic, the role of the military in pandemic response was extended to facilitating surveillance of citizens.[25] Framing of "securitization," however, to some extent, can be seen as a form of "threat" to citizens. For instance, the governments can justify the imposition of a political emergency during a pandemic that could potentially bring further harm to the civic space in the long term.[26] Risk and insecurity, anxiety, and unease are increasingly salient factors in defining the nature of political community, the meaning of citizenship, the way states govern, and how citizens govern themselves. Therefore, framing the politics concerning security is always a dangerous move, not least because security and insecurity are mutually reinforcing concepts.[27]

Findings

The data collected are organized in three different tables, namely the EIU Democracy Index, the CIVICUS civic space index, and the author's own compilation between 2018 and 2021.

The Economist Intelligence Unit (EIU) Democracy Index in Table 5.1 shows the performance of the five countries under the study. The Democracy Index is based on five categories: electoral process and pluralism; civil liberties; the functioning of government; political participation; and political culture. Based on their scores on 60 indicators within these categories, each country is classified as one of four types of regimes: full democracy, flawed democracy, hybrid regime, and authoritarian regime. From the EIU Democracy Index from 2018 to 2020, all four countries, namely Indonesia, Malaysia, the Philippines, and Singapore are under the category of flawed democracy except Brunei that does not have any data available. Flawed democracies in this context of the EIU refer to countries that are not full democracies (scores greater than 6 or lesser than 8). Looking at the patterns and trends between 2018 and 2020, Malaysia is the only country that has shown some progress towards democratization, from 6.88 in 2018 to 7.19 in 2020. This is also reflected in political change, evident in the country after a peaceful regime change since 2018. The triumph of *Pakatan Harapan* as the opposition allowed Tun Mahathir Mohamad to be re-elected as the

Table 5.1 EIU index

| Country | Democracy Index (EIU) | | | |
	2018[28]	2019[29]	2020[30]	2021
Brunei	-	-	-	-
Indonesia	6.39	6.48	6.30	-
	Flawed democracy	Flawed democracy	Flawed democracy	
Malaysia	6.88	7.16	7.19	-
	Flawed democracy	Flawed democracy	Flawed democracy	
Philippines	6.71 Flawed democracy	6.64	6.56	-
		Flawed democracy	Flawed democracy	
Singapore	6.38	6.02	6.03	-
	Flawed democracy	Flawed democracy	Flawed democracy	

Source: EIU

Table 5.2 CIVICUS Civic Space Index

Country	Civic Space Index			
	2018[31]	*2019[32]*	*2020[33]*	*2021[34]*
Brunei	Obstructed	Repressed	Repressed	Repressed
Indonesia	Obstructed	Obstructed	Obstructed	Obstructed
Malaysia	Obstructed	Obstructed	Obstructed	Obstructed
Philippines	Obstructed	Obstructed	Repressed	Repressed
Singapore	Obstructed	Obstructed	Obstructed	Repressed

Source: CIVICUS Monitor

prime minister. Malaysia's ability to achieve an impressive leap in its democracy occurred along with a regime change.

Table 5.2 shows the civic space index released by the CIVICUS Monitor, a research tool that provides data on the state of civil society and civic freedoms in 196 countries. The data disaggregates countries' civic space into five categories: closed, repressed, obstructed, narrowed, or open. Southeast Asian nations in general, have experienced a broad and continued contraction of the political space and civil liberties over the past 4 years. For the Philippines, it was under the category of obstructed from 2018 to 2019. The CIVICUS monitor downgraded Philippines to repressed in 2020 due to the vilification of activists and targeting of human rights defenders and journalists. Although Brunei has been in the category of obstructed in 2018, the CIVICUS monitor downgraded the country to repressed in 2019 due to curtailed civic freedoms, censorship of the media, and revision of the *Sharia* (Islamic penal code) that imposes the death sentence for various offenses.

Table 5.3 depicts extant movement control restrictions of varying degrees that are evident in the management of COVID-19 in the five countries. While it is generally accepted to some extent that there can be some form of restriction in exercising civil and political rights during a pandemic, there are many elements of depriving civic space and freedom at the expense of a health crisis, as evident in the data collection. Much of the recent Southeast Asian repression has been justified on the grounds of the pandemic which has provided cover for the introduction of extraordinary powers. While these are theoretically legitimate responses to a severe public health crisis, many nations have restricted legitimate political expression. In line with the research aim, the chapter will only focus on legislation that impacts the functioning of civic space.

COVID-19 legislative measures across Brunei, Indonesia, Malaysia, the Philippines, and Singapore intended to deter and prosecute the spread of disinformation through social media and to silence critics of the state. Activists are concerned about the vagueness of fake news laws across Southeast Asia and their implications of its use on freedom of expression and opinion in states with increasing human rights concerns.

Table 5.3 Measures on COVID-19

Country	Measures on COVID-19
Brunei	**Public Order Act.**[35]
	Infectious Diseases Act, Chapter 204.[36]
Indonesia	**State of Emergency.**[37] First declaration: 28 February 2020 Initial timespan of decree: 2 weeks Revoked/ Ended on/ Renewed until: Renewed and ended on 29 May
	Electronic Information and Transactions (ITE) Law.[38]
	Implementation of massive restrictions (PSBB).[39] - Regulation No. 33 of 2020 and Decree No. 380 of 2020
Malaysia	**Development in COVID-19 Measures:** March 2020: Movement Control Order April 2020: Extension of Movement Control Order May 2020: Conditional Movement Control Order June 2020: Recovery Movement Control Order January 2021: State of Emergency June 2021: National Recovery Plan
Philippines	**Prevention and Control of Infectious Diseases Act 1988.**[40] **State of Public Health Emergency** First declaration: 9 March 2020 Initial timespan of decree: 3 months Ended on: 8 June.[41] **State of Calamity** First declaration: 16 March 2020 Initial Timespan of Decree: 6 months Renewed until 13 September 2021.[42]
	Bayanihan to Heal as One Act First declaration: 23 March 2020 Initial Timespan of Decree: 3 months Ended on: 24 June 2020
	Bayanihan to Recover as One Act (Bayanihan 2).[43] Information: officially designated as Republic Act No. 11494 First declaration: September 2020
Singapore	**COVID-19 (Temporary Measures) Act 2020.**[44]
	Revised Supplementary Supply (FY 2020) Act 2020.[45]
	Parliamentary Elections (COVID-19 Special Arrangements) Act 2020.[46]
	Constitution of the Republic of Singapore (Amendment) Act 2020.[47]
	COVID-19 (Temporary Measures for Solemnization and Registration of Marriages) Act 2020.[48]

Source: Author's own compilation

Brunei is an absolute monarchy. The country's only television station is state-run and its journalists often practice self-censorship.[49] The Sultanate has been downgraded from obstructed to repressed since 2019 due to the curtailment of civic and media freedoms. In Brunei, under Section 34 in Chapter 148 of the Public Order Act, anyone who circulates "fake news" on social media can be fined up to US$2,100 or imprisoned up to 36 months.[50] In one instance, Hajah Faizah Haji Abdul Gapar was charged under Section 34, of the Public Order Act, Chapter 148 for a video recording which contained a false statement.[51] As a COVID-19 precautionary measure, Brunei had instituted mass-testing since January 2020 and implemented travel bans in and out of the Sultanate since March 15, 2020.[52] Furthermore, the Sultanate introduced BruHealth—an online tracking application introduced on May 16, 2020—for tracing infected COVID-19 cases and their contacts. The development of BruHealth is outsourced to a Chinese company, Yidu Cloud Technology.[53] Although the Minister of Finance and Economy, Dr Amin Yiew, reassured citizens that the tracking application was a credible news source, there were concerns that privacy of citizens could be compromised.

Indonesia declared a state of emergency on February 28, 2020. A few public health emergency decrees were declared. For instance, the provisions of the Public Health Emergency (Decree 11/2020) imposed a ban on large-scale social gatherings, made masking mandatory, and imposed penalties on the circulation of fake news on social media. Individuals who did not conform to the masking in public were subjected to community service, a measure aimed at public shaming.[54] Massive restrictions under the Indonesian Large-scale Social Restrictions or *Pembatasan Sosial Berskala Besar di Indonesia* (PSBB) were also implemented under the Regulation No.33 of 2020 and Decree No.380 of 2020.[55] PSBB was a provisional measure taken by central and provincial governments to restrict mass gatherings within a city or province—similar to a semi-lockdown. Apart from the PSBB, the government implemented the 2008 Electronic Information and Transactions Law to curtail individuals critical of the government's handling of the pandemic and "fake news."[56]

Malaysia is the only country that has shown a relative improvement in its democracy index from 2018 to 2020, mainly due to the political change in the country that ended the 61-year uninterrupted rule of the *Barisan Nasional* (National Front). Since the pandemic first struck Malaysia, the country's politics have been highly contentious and debated. Several temporary measures were enacted, such as various phases of the Movement Control Order that is being put in place since March 2020, and a State of Emergency was also declared in January 2021.[57] Two legislations that were contested within Malaysia for the restrictions imposed on civic space included the Emergency (Prevention and Control of Infectious Diseases Amendment Ordinance 2021) and the Emergency (Essential Powers No. 2, Ordinance 2021). A few protests took place in Malaysia during the pandemic. For instance, there are a series of #Lawan protests organized by the youths under Sekretariat Solidariti Rakyat (SSR). The SSR previously organized several small protests, including the "Black Flag" protest at Dataran Merdeka on July 17, 2020 and a vehicle convoy on July 24, 2020. It is a series of protests to demand the resignation of the then prime minister Muhyiddin Yassin, a full Parliament sitting, and a moratorium on the repayment of all loans.

Some also brought mock corpses wrapped in *kapan* cloth to symbolize the high number of daily deaths from COVID-19 in Malaysia and the inadequacies of the healthcare system in coping with the challenges of COVID-19.[58]

In July 2020, Al-Jazeera in its investigative documentary "Locked Up in Malaysia's Lockdown" contended that while efforts to contain the pandemic were successful, the Malaysian government took advantage of the Movement Control Order to crackdown on undocumented migrant workers and refugees.[59] On January 30, 2020, the Malaysian government announced that migrant/undocumented migrant workers or refugees who were suspected of testing positive for COVID-19 or who were in close contact with COVID-19 cases were exempt from paying outpatient fees at government hospitals.[60] But on the eve of Labor Day (May 1, 2020), hundreds of undocumented migrant workers and refugees were arrested in a massive raid operation near Jalan Masjid India, Kuala Lumpur. A few weeks later, in Klang valley, Selayang and Gombak, thousands of undocumented workers were rounded-up in immigration detention centers.[61] The chain of events and responses made by the Malaysian government since the first Movement Control Order was introduced reveal the lack of coordination and consistency between different levels of government in handling the problems of migrant workers.

The Philippines has an uneven trajectory of building democratic institutions. Three-and-a-half decades after the 1986 People Power Revolution put an end to Ferdinand Marcos' dictatorship, the country appears to have developed an electoral habit of rotating power between populist and reformist presidents.[62] The government's response to the pandemic had been incrementally securitized, with strong parallels to President Duterte's violent war on drugs.[63] In April 2020, 32 people were arrested and charged for spreading "fake news" about the COVID-19 pandemic on social media.[64] Human rights defenders involved in food distribution in Bulacan Province were charged with violating the "Bayanihan to Heal as One" Act that gives authorization to all government agencies and local government units to enforce disease control prevention measures and to enhance community quarantine. The Philippine government accused human rights defenders of "sedition" after newspapers with anti-government content were found in their vehicle.[65] The Philippine government has relied on influential military figures in its COVID-19 response.

By August 2020, the Philippines, already under quarantine measures involving shuttered businesses, enforced curfew hours, and restricted supplies, was at a crossroads. Overwhelmed by rapidly-filling ICUs amidst spiraling COVID-19 cases, the country's healthcare professionals called for time-out measures to restrict movements and reduce infections with a view to buy time and plan forward in the management of the pandemic.[66] They insisted that President Duterte enforce 2 weeks of stricter lockdowns and militarized checkpoints. Between August 2020 and August 2021, the Philippines remained in one of the longest-running strictest quarantines, with restrictions on movement that risked fines or beatings from the law enforcement agencies if broken. Those Filipinos arrested for violating movement restrictions were compelled to do hard physical labor or confined to cells that increased their vulnerability to the virus.[67] The see-sawing of movement restrictions disproportionately affected daily wage-earners, comprising nearly 38% of the nearly 110 million Filipinos who would be tagged as quarantine violators.

The Philippine Anti-Terror Act (2020) and a militarized COVID-19 approach of the Duterte administration enhanced violence towards health workers. For example, in 2020, Mary Rose Sancelan, a city health officer in Negros Oriental, and the only doctor serving in the province's COVID-19 pandemic response, was shot dead with her husband. She was previously red-tagged by a local anti-communist vigilante group. In December, 2021, Raul Andutan, a surgeon and medical director in Cagayan De Oro, was killed in broad daylight for a reported bounty of US$3000.[68] The Alliance of Health Workers, a local healthcare union was accused of fronting the Communist Party of the Philippines.[69] Amidst the pandemic incidents such as the eviction of nurses from properties for fear that they tested COVID-positive, the government was compelled to pass the Mandatory Protection of Health Workers, Frontliners, and Patients Act. The Philippine government is fearful that continued assaults on health personnel would create medical deserts, depriving entire communities of healthcare.[70]

By April 2021, the Philippines had one of the worst COVID outbreaks in Southeast Asia. The country's shortcomings in the management of COVID-19 are largely attributable to the country's limited investment in healthcare and insufficient health personnel that resulted in delayed contact tracing and mass testing and overwhelmed hospitals.[71]

Among the five countries of maritime Southeast Asia, Singapore's response to the COVID-19 crisis has won international plaudits with its adequate healthcare and vaccination program. The country's highly centralized approach to policymaking, easy access to the residents' private data, as well as the harsh penalties for breaches of COVID regulations reflect the direct costs that come with the securitization approach. After the city state detected the first case of COVID on January 2, 2020, the Ministry of Health instituted temperature screenings of incoming passengers, issued mandatory stay-at-home orders to residents returning from China, and undertook aggressive testing of the population. Between January and early-March 2020, during its first wave, Singapore had among the lowest case-fatality rates in the world attributed to COVID-19.[72] But, COVID-19 cases leapfrogged tenfold from 100 to 1000 between March 1 and 30, 2020. Soon after a COVID-19 outbreak was recorded in the country's dormitories housing foreign workers around late-March 2020, the government implemented extensive testing of dormitory workers, segregation of sick from healthy workers, and on-site healthcare facilities.

Between March 20 and the first week of June, the city state introduced circuit-breaking measures and partial lockdowns and implemented the Protection from Online Falsehoods and Manipulation Act to tackle coronavirus-related misinformation. Furthermore, the government in collaboration with Singapore United unveiled *TraceTogether*, a mobile application that deploys Bluetooth technology to track COVID-19 cases and their contacts. As Hallam Stevens and Monamie Bhadra Haines contend:

> Rather than linking people together via a network, the phone becomes a sensor through which to detect an invisible enemy in the body of another individual. In fact, the only way people can ultimately be "linked" is via the centralized authority (that is, when the Ministry of Health requests or requires contact tracing). The government remains the obligatory passage point in the network.[73]

The *TraceTogether* application mobilizes the rhetoric of citizen science and democratic participation. However, Media Studies Scholars have raised ethical concerns related to privacy protection of citizens' data and the conduct of surveillance in a panoptic and auto-regulatory society that privileges socio-political discipline.[74]

A comparison between the EIU Democracy Index (5.1) and the CIVICUS Civic Space Index indicates that the scores do not correlate directly to how open the state is. In other words, the state is not the only factor to understand the effect of COVID-19 on civic space. For instance, Singapore is downgraded from obstructed to repressed by the CIVICUS Monitor. However, its management of the COVID-19 pandemic has been widely praised. One argument could be due to Singapore's close relationship between the party and the state that gives it substantial infrastructural power to manage the health crisis.[75]

Discussion

Having analyzed COVID-19 across the five countries in the maritime Southeast Asia, it is inevitable to conclude that securitization is the underlining feature of state response to the coronavirus crisis. Securitization of the pandemic was reinforced with a narrative characterizing the state's situation as being at war against an "unseen enemy."[76]

Before COVID-19 emerged in early 2020, the Southeast Asian region was already characterized by high levels of inequality and low levels of social protection. How does the COVID-19 response impact politics, including democracy and human rights in Southeast Asia? The COVID era has seen an onslaught on human rights and democratic norms by the authorities across the region. Based on the data above, the five countries examined have used pandemics to curb already shrinking civic space. In the name of enforcing pandemic-necessitated lockdowns and shutdowns, most governments have invoked emergency clauses to curb civil rights.

There are five novel findings as observed in this chapter, with the focus on their impact on civic space. First, it is observed that most containment measures, as shown in Table 5.3, have been enacted under existing national disaster management or public health emergency legislation without necessarily a specific reference to human rights or the scrutiny required for the official declaration of a state of emergency. In some circumstances, questions have been raised on the application of emergency measures, including whether they meet the requirements of necessity, proportionality, non-discrimination, and adherence to international legal norms. Vaguely worded provisions without necessary safeguards and limitations can potentially restrict the rights to information, privacy, and freedom of movement, expression, association, peaceful assembly, and asylum. In some cases, there are no safeguards such as sunset or review clauses to ensure a return to ordinary laws as soon as the emergency is over. It will therefore be essential to review their application in line with international human rights law.

Second, the cases of increasing legal restrictions imposed on civic activities and defamation and criminalization of human rights defenders and democracy advocates in the pretext for physical distancing and social control to combat COVID-19 is a concerning trend about the shrinking civic space as illustrated. This includes the usage of various legislations targeting misinformation and disinformation under the label of "fake news," that has affected the enjoyment of freedom of thought, opinions and expression, and assembly and association. There is also concern about the arbitrary application of the rule-of-law principle under the state of emergency and administrative erosion of democratic rights. Apart from that, there is also concern about the worsening human rights situation under the pretext of countering COVID-19 as reported, such as harassment on human rights defenders, particularly in the Philippines. Linking to that, there is no evidence that harsh policies in the Philippines produce a more effective pandemic response.

Third, advances toward democracy in Southeast Asia, that came at an immense cost, are at risk of being steadily eroded. Historically, both Indonesia and the Philippines can be considered amongst the most vibrant democracies of Southeast Asia. However, the EIU Democracy Index in Table 5.1 and the CIVICUS Civic Space Index in Table 5.2 have revealed otherwise. The indexes have shown that the reality is more complex. Formal democratic institutions coexist with endemic corruption and cronyism in both nations, enmeshed with weak political institutions and turgid state bureaucracies. In recent years, this has helped pave the way for Rodrigo Duterte in the Philippines and Joko Widodo in Indonesia. Their administrations have downplayed scientific evidence related to COVID-19. This further indicates how the securitization approach on COVID-19 can also produce negative consequences on civic space. The COVID-19 pandemic has put Joko Widodo's second-term into a challenging period. For instance, his prioritization of economy over public health, and neglect of commitments to uphold or strengthen an array of political and civil rights that are critical to the health of Indonesian democracy have received some setbacks.[77]

Fourth, the EIU Democracy Index and CIVICUS Civic Space Index related to civic space on issues such as freedom of assembly, freedom of movement, and freedom of expression have generally shown that the response to and the management of COVID-19 across the five countries are varied. They do not correlate directly to how democratic or how open a country is. Almost all countries except Malaysia have revealed a regression of democracy. Similarly, it is observed that a better position for Malaysia in the EIU Democracy Index does not automatically translate into improvement in civil liberties. The declining trend of democracy in Southeast Asia has shown that civil liberties, as one of the variables in the index, are consistently situated at the lowest rank. As observed, the EIU Democracy Index reflects the link where the absence of adequate civic spaces would threaten democracy and peace. Governments actively constrain civic spaces across the region in multiple ways, including new cyber-security legislation and older legislative frameworks with punitive consequences. There are numerous overlapping restrictions on freedom of speech and action throughout the region. COVID-19 is making this worse from the declining index scores as shown in EIU Democracy Index and the CIVICUS Civic Space Index.

Fifth, the spread of COVID-19 is potentially accelerating autocratization across these five countries. Leaders have used the pandemic as a pretext to consolidate their power through Emergency decrees, curfews, or similar laws in countries such as the Philippines. However, such laws have also been used to crack down on government critics and undermine opposition parties, furthering authoritarian power grab. The COVID-19 pandemic developing in this context is seen as a threat to individual humans and is assessed as a threat that could endanger the survival of society.[78]

Conclusion

COVID-19 in Southeast Asia has highlighted the strengths and weaknesses of a regional approach to the pandemic. The weakness of the ASEAN-led approach to the pandemic could be attributed to the fragmented nature of its health sector. The outbreaks of SARS and H5N1 Avian Influenza across the region highlighted the need for intergovernmental coordination, not only among ASEAN health ministries but also across government agencies. As a response to the SARS outbreak, regional health platforms such as ASEAN Emergency Operations Center Network for Public Health or EOC were developed. The early ASEAN response to COVID-19 was swift. On January 4, 2020—when the regional group received notification of unexplained pneumonia clusters in Wuhan—the EOC was activated during the pandemic to provide daily situational updates.

Despite responding rapidly to the pandemic in early 2020, ASEAN economies have been hit by the ripple effects of COVID-19. The region relies heavily on tourism, manufacturing, international trade, and intra-regional migration. Apart from the health crisis, member states of ASEAN witnessed economic disruption. The disruption resulted from localized lockdowns in Indonesia and the Philippines, and the Movement Control Order in Malaysia to closed international borders in Indonesia and Singapore that had an adverse impact on peoples' livelihoods.

Recognizing the importance of a regional approach to the pandemic, the ASEAN Secretariat's Socio-Cultural Community Department partnered with the Asia Foundation, the Rockefeller Foundation, and the Australian government to conduct a rapid assessment of the fallout of the pandemic on peoples' livelihoods across the ten member states of the ASEAN.[79] The study noted that the pandemic threatens to increase economic inequality and upend the region's two-decade progress in reversing poverty. Given the significant contribution of intra-regional labor migration to Southeast Asia, ASEAN member states could do more to protect migrant workers, not only those who remain in their host country but also those who return to their homes. Promoting the economic integration of informal and intra-regional migrant workers requires a coordinated regional strategy that involves the ministries of social welfare, labor, health, and immigration of the ASEAN member states.

However, ASEAN's multilateral response to the COVID-19 pandemic is circumscribed by its efforts to promote regional integration rather than a supranational union of states where members cede aspects of sovereignty to the regional grouping. The ASEAN's principle of "non-interference" and national sovereignty of member states limits fully-integrated cross-border response to the pandemic.[80] The region's lack of a cohesive regional response to COVID-19 remains a continuous challenge that should be clearly addressed. In retrospect, the securitization of a non-traditional threat such as COVID-19 may be necessary for a government to control the pandemic. However, the findings show that the countries examined legitimize extraordinary actions to cope with a crisis. The securitization approach is observed in the five countries at the expense of civic rights and freedom, and prolongation of authoritarianism.[81] One significant piece of evidence is the usage of legislation in curbing media freedom under the name of misinformation and disinformation on COVID-19. This reflects the use of selective securitization to achieve a discursive hegemony aimed at controlling the information about the pandemic.

Acknowledgments

This work was supported by Universiti Malaya (UM) under GPF035A-2020. The author would like to sincerely appreciate the contribution of her research assistant, Jessie Lee, in completing this work. I would like to thank Dr Vivek Neelakantan for his thorough editorial feedback that improved the overall quality of the chapter.

Notes

1　Katherine Putz, Abhignan Rej, Sebastian Strangio and Shannon Tiezzi, "How COVID-19 Changed Asia," *The Diplomat*, March 12, 2021, https://thediplomat.com/2021/03/how-covid-19-changed-asia/.

2　Larry Diamond, "Democracy versus the Pandemic: The Coronavirus is Emboldening Autocrats the World Over," *Foreign Affairs*, June 13, 2020, https://www.foreignaffairs.com/articles/world/2020-06-13/democracy-versus-pandemic.

3　S. Repucci, and A. Slipowitz, "Democracy under Lockdown: The Impact of COVID-19 on the Global struggle for freedom," *Freedom House* 2020, https://freedomhouse.org/report/special-report/2020/democracy-under-lockdown; A. E. Yamin, and R. Habibi, "Human Rights and Coronavirus: What's at Stake for Truth, Trust, and Democracy," *Health and Human Rights Journal* (March 1, 2020); C. Valerio, "Human Rights and Covid-19 Pandemic," *JBRA Assisted Reproduction* 24, no. 3 (2020): 379.

4　See Vivek Neelakantan, "History of Pandemics in Southeast Asia: A Return of National Anxieties," *ISIS Current Bibliography* v. 3 (2021), https://isiscb.org/special-issue-on-pandemics/essay.html?essayID=01.

5　Sara Davis, *Containing Contagion: The Politics of Disease Outbreaks in Southeast Asia* (Baltimore: Johns Hopkins University Press), 4.

6　See for e.g., Marie Lamy and Kai Hong Phua, "Southeast Asian Cooperation in Health: A Comparative Perspective on Regional Health governance in ASEAN and the EU," *Asia Europe Journal* 10 (2012): 233–50.

7　For details refer Edward Aspinall, *Opposing Suharto: Compromise, Resistance and Regime Change in Indonesia* (Stanford: Stanford University Press, 2005).

8　Aurel Croissant and Jeffrey Haynes, "Democratic Regression in Asia: Introduction," *Democratization* 28, no. 1 (2021): 1–21. For the Malaysian context, refer Sheila Nair, "The Limits of Protest and Prospects for Political Reform in Malaysia," *Critical Asian Studies* 39, no. 3 (2007): 339–68.

9　Jürgen Rüland, "Covid-19 and ASEAN: Strengthening State-Centrism, Eroding Inclusiveness, Testing Cohesion," *The International Spectator* 56, no. 2 (2021): 72–92.

10　Khoo Ying Hooi, "Southeast Asia's Pandemic Politics and Human Rights: Trends and Lessons," *LSE*, October 1, 2020, https://blogs.lse.ac.uk/seac/2020/10/01/southeast-asias-pandemic-politics-and-human-rights-trends-and-lessons/.

11　For a conceptual understanding of the operationalization of biopolitics during the times of coronavirus see Christopher J. Lee, "The Necropolitics of COVID-19," *Africa is a Country Blog*, April 1, 2020, https://africasacountry.com/2020/04/the-necropolitics-of-covid-19. For a comprehensive understanding of the Asian context see S. Sornbanlang, "The Securitization of the Coronavirus in Asian Countries: A Paradox of National Security and Human Security During the COVID-19 Crisis," in *Global Security in Times of Covid-19: New Security Challenges*, C. Varin edited (Palgrave MacMillan: Cham, 2022), 145–70. For the international context see for e.g. Jessica Kirk, "The Politics of Exceptionalism: Securitization and COVID-19," *Global Studies Quarterly* 1 (2021): 1–12. Kirk contends that dominant conceptions of securitization as an elite-driven process, in which leaders point to an existential threat to justify exceptional responses, are not necessarily borne out in practice.

12　John Morrissey, "Planetary Precarity and 'More-Than-Human Security': The Securitization Challenge in the Aftermath of COVID-19," *Journal of Human Security* 17, no. 1 (2021): 15–22, DOI: 1112924/johs2021.17010015

13　Ibid.

14　For a basic understanding of securitization during the COVID-19 pandemic see D. Duarte and Marcelo Valença "Securitising COVID-19: The Limits of the Copenhagen School," *Contexto Internacional* 43, no. 2 (May–August 2021): 235–57; For the Indonesian context refer Chairil, Tangguh, "Indonesian Government's COVID-19 Measures, January–May 2020: Late Response and Public Health Securitization," *Jurnal Ilmu Sosial dan Ilmu Politik* 24, no. 2 (2020): 128–52, doi: 10.22146/jsp.55863.

15 Barry Buzan, Ole Wæver, and Jaap De Wilde. *Security: A New Framework for Analysis* (London: Lynne Rienner Publishers, 1998).

16 Ibid. See also Supalak Ganjanakhundee, "COVID-19 in Thailand: The Securitization of a Non-traditional Threat," *ISEAS Yusof Ishak Perspective* 51 (May 22, 2020), https://www.iseas.edu.sg/wp-content/uploads/2020/03/ISEAS_Perspective_2020_51.pdf.

17 Michaela Grančayová, "Plagues of Egypt – The COVID-19 Crisis and the Role of Securitization Dilemmas in the Authoritarian Regime Survival Strategies in Egypt and Turkey, *Czech Journal of International Relations* (2021), DOI: 10.32422/mv.1766.

18 J. A. Vouri, "Illocutionary Logic and Strands of Securitization: Applying the Theory of Securitization to the Study of Non-democratic Political Orders," *European Journal of International Relations* 14, no. 1 (2008): 65–99.

19 Stefan Elbe, *Security and Global Health: Toward the Medicalization of Insecurity* (UK: Polity Press, 2010). See also Jiyong Jin and Joe Thomas Karackattu, "Infectious Diseases Securitization and WHO's Dilemma," *Biosecurity and Bioterrorism: Biodefense Strategy, Practice, and Science* 9, no. 2 (2011), DOI: 10.1089/bsp.2010.0045.

20 Colin McInnes and Simon Rushton, "HIV/AIDS and Securitization Theory," *European Journal of International Relations* 19, no. 1 (2012): 115–38. For SARS refer Adam Kamradt-Scott, *Managing Global Health Security: The World Health Organization and Disease Outbreak Control* (Basingstoke: Palgrave MacMillan, 2015), 79–100. For Ebola and Zika refer Deisy de Freitas Lima Ventura, "From Ebola to Zika: International Emergencies and the Securitization of Global Health," *Cadernos de Saúde Pública* 32, no. 4 (2016), DOI: https://doi.org/10.1590/0102-311X00033316.

21 Stephane Baele, "On the Securitization of COVID-19," *Pandemipolitics.net*, April 9, 2020, https://pandemipolitics.net/baele/.

22 Tangguh Chairil. "Indonesian Government's COVID-19 Measures, January–May 2020: Late Response and Public Health Securitization," *Jurnal Ilmu Sosial dan Ilmu Politik* 24, no. 2 (2020): 128–52, DOI: 10.22146/jsp.55863.

23 Ibid.

24 Alexander Wendt and Michael Barnett, "Dependent State Formation and Third World Militarization," *Review of International Studies* 19 (1993): 321–47. See also J. W. Schofield, "Increasing the Generalizability of Qualitative Research," in *The Qualitative Researcher's Companion,* A.Michael Huberman and Matthew Miles edited (Thousand Oaks, CA: Sage, 2002).

25 For the Thai context, see for e.g., Piyapong Boossabong and Pobsook Chamchong, "Coping with COVID-19 in a Non-Democratic System: Policy Lessons from Thailand's Centralised Government," *International Review of Public Policy* 2, no.3 (2020): 358–71.

26 See also Felix S Bethke and Jonas Wolff, "COVID-19 and Shrinking Civic Spaces: Patterns and Consequences," *Zeitschrift für Friedens-und Konfliktforschung* 9, no. 2 (2020): 363–74.

27 Ibid.

28 The Economist Intelligence Unit, "Democracy Index 2018: Me too? Political Participation, Protest and Democracy," *The Economist Intelligence Unit* (2019): 24.

29 The Economist Intelligence Unit, "Democracy Index 2019: A Year of Demo-
    cratic Setbacks and Popular Protest," *The Economist Intelligence Unit* (2020):
    26.
30 The Economist Intelligence Unit, "Democracy Index 2020: In sickness and in
    health?" *The Economist Intelligence Unit* (2021): 29.
31 CIVICUS, "People Power Under Attack," *CIVICUS* (2019), https://civicus.
    org/documents/GlobalCIVICUSMonitorReport.2019.pdf.
32 Ibid.
33 CIVICUS, "People Power Under Attack 2020," *CIVICUS* (2020), https://
    civicus.contentfiles.net/media/assets/file/GlobalReport2020.pdf.
34 CIVICUS, "CIVICUS Monitor: Tracking Civic Space," *CIVICUS* (2021),
    https://www.civicus.org/index.php/what-we-do/innovate/civicus-monitor.
35 Asia Centre, "Defending Freedom of Expression," *Asia Centre* (2020), https://
    asiacentre.org/wp-content/uploads/Defending_Freedom_of_Expression_
    Fake_News_Laws_in_East_and_Southeast_Asia.pdf.
36 Ministry of Health Brunei Darussalam, "Directives Under the Infectious
    Diseases Act Chapter 204," http://www.moh.gov.bn/SitePages/Arahan-Ara-
    han%20di%20bawah%20BAB%2062A%20Akta%20Penyakit%20Berjang-
    kit%20Penggal%20204.aspx.
37 Asia Centre, "COVID-19 and Democracy in Southeast Asia," *Asia Centre*
    (2020), https://asiacentre.org/wp-content/uploads/COVID-19-and-Democracy-
    in-Southeast-Asia-Building-Resilience-Fighting-Authoritarianism.pdf.
38 Abdurrachman Satrio, "State of Emergency Through the Back Door,"
    Verfassungsblog, April 21, 2020, https://verfassungsblog.de/state-of-
    emergency-through-the-back-door/.
39 Kresna Panggabean, Jeremiah Purba, Salman Sembiring, "COVID-19:
    Legal Update on Employment Law issues in Indonesia as a Result of
    Implementation of PSBB," *Norton Rose Fulbright,* April 2020, https://www.
    nortonrosefulbright.com/fr-ca/centre-du-savoir/publications/3449b9f2/
    covid-19-legal-update-on-employment-law-issues-in-indonesia.
40 Wei Liang Tan and Tai Kean Lynn, "Covid-19: Emergency Ordinance
    2021 Gazetted," *Skrine*, March 2, 2021, https://www.skrine.com/insights/
    covid-19-updates/covid-19-emergency-prevention-and-control-of-infec.
41 Asia Centre, "COVID-19 and Democracy in Southeast Asia," Second time the
    work is cited.
42 Wei Liang Tan and Tai Kean Lynn, "Covid-19: Emergency Ordinance
    2021 Gazetted," *Skrine*, March 2, 2021, https://www.skrine.com/insights/
    covid-19-updates/covid-19-emergency-prevention-and-control-of-infec.
43 Merez, Arianne, "Duterte signs Bayanihan 2 into law," *ABS-CBN*,
    September 11, 2020, https://news.abs-cbn.com/news/09/11/20/duterte-signs-
    bayanihan-2-into-law.
44 Republic of Singapore, "Covid-19 (Temporary Measures) Act 2020," *Republic
    of Singapore*, April 9, 2020, https://sso.agc.gov.sg/Act/COVID19TMA2020.
45 Republic of Singapore, "Revised Supplementary Supply (FY 2020) Act
    2020," *Republic of Singapore*, April 7, 2020, https://www.parliament.gov.
    sg/docs/default-source/default-document-library/revised-supplementary-
    supply-(fy-2020)-bill-20-2020.pdf.
46 Republic of Singapore, "Parliamentary Elections (COVID-19 Special
    Arrangements) Act 2020," *Republic of Singapore,* May 29, 2020, https://sso.
    agc.gov.sg/Act/PECOVID19SAA2020.
    Republic of Singapore, "Constitution of the Republic of Singapore (Amend-
    ment) Act 2020," *Republic of Singapore,* May 22, 2020, https://sso.agc.gov.sg/
    Acts-Supp/22-2020/Published/20200520.

47 Ibid.
48 Republic of Singapore, "COVID-19 (Temporary Measures for Solemnization and Registration of Marriages) Act 2020," *Republic of Singapore*, May 22, 2020, https://sso.agc.gov.sg/Act/COVID19TMSRMA2020.
49 C. L. J Li, "The Cyberspace in Brunei," *Asian Politics & Policy* 4, no. 1 (2012): 127–31.
50 Asia Centre, "Defending Freedom of Expression," *Asia Centre* (2020), https://asiacentre.org/wp-content/uploads/Defending_Freedom_of_Expression_Fake_News_Laws_in_East_and_Southeast_Asia.pdf.
51 RTB News, "Public Order Act," BruDirect.Com, September 29, 2021, https://www.brudirect.com/news.php?id=128717. In the video recording, the defendant made an unsubstantiated claim that a restaurant in Mabohai had been discovered by the police to be operating with employees who were in violation of their Quarantine Orders.
52 See Riyanti Djalante, Laely Nurhidayah, Hoang Van Minh et al., "Review and Analysis of Current Responses to COVID-19 in Indonesia: Period of January to March 2020," *Progress in Disaster Science* 6 (2020), DOI: https://doi.org/10.1016/j.pdisas.2020.100091.
53 Li Li Pang, "Leadership and Crisis Communication During COVID-19: The Case of Brunei Darussalam," *Policy and Governance Review* 5, no. 2 (2021): 97–112.
54 Asia Centre, "The Securitisation of COVID-19 Health Protocols: Policing the Vulnerable, Infringing their Rights," *Asia Centre* (2021), https://asiacentre.org/wp-content/uploads/The-Securitisation-of-COVID-19-Health-Protocols-Policing-the-Vulnerable-Infringing-their-Rights.pdf.
55 Kresna Panggabean, Jeremiah Purba, and Salman Sembiring, "COVID-19: Legal Update on Employment Law issues in Indonesia as a Result of Implementation of PSBB," *Norton Rose Fulbright,* April 2020, https://www.nortonrosefulbright.com/fr-ca/centre-du-savoir/publications/3449b9f2/covid-19-legal-update-on-employment-law-issues-in-indonesia.
56 Asia Centre, "Defending Freedom of Expression," *Asia Centre* (2020), https://asiacentre.org/wp-content/uploads/Defending_Freedom_of_Expression_Fake_News_Laws_in_East_and_Southeast_Asia.pdf.
57 Istana Negara, "Kenyataan Media," *Istana Negara*, January 12, 2021.
58 Mohamad Saim, Atiqah Bt Mohamed, "Dalam Mahkamah Majistret di Kuala Lumpur Dalam Wilayah Persekutuan Kuala Lumpur Permohonan Jenayah No: WA-89-939-08/2021," *Makhamah Majistret Kuala Lumpur*, August 20, 2021.
59 Asia Centre, "The Securitisation of COVID-19 Health Protocols."
60 Andika Wahab, "The Outbreak of COVID-19 in Malaysia: Pushing Migrant Workers at the Margin," *Social Sciences and Humanities Open* 2 (2020): 100073, DOI: https://doi.org/10.1016/j.ssaho.2020.100073.
61 Ibid.
62 Mesrob Vartavarian, "Rodrigo Duterte and the Philippine Presidency: Rupture or Legitimacy?", *IIAS Newsletter* 80 (Summer 2018), https://www.iias.asia/the-newsletter/article/rodrigo-duterte-philippine-presidency-rupture-or-cyclicity.
63 Asia Centre, "Waging War Against COVID-19: The Securitisation of the Health Response in Five Asian Countries," *Asia Centre* (2021), https://asiacentre.org/wp-content/uploads/Briefing-Note-Waging-War-Against-COVID-19.pdf.
64 CNN Philippines Staff, "32 arrested over 'fake' COVID-19 News," *CNN Philippines*, April 6, 2020, https://www.cnnphilippines.com/news/2020/4/6/arrests-over-coronavirus-fake-news.html.

65 Baysa-Barredo, Joel Mark, "Problematizing the Securitization of Covid-19 in Southeast Asia: A Necessary Step Towards an Inclusive, Rights-Centred Normal," *SHAPE-SEA,* June 16, 2020, https://shapesea.com/op-ed/problematizing-the-securitization-of-covid-19-in-southeast-asia-a-necessary-step-towards-an-inclusive-rights-centred-normal/.
66 Patricia Denise M. Chiu, "Why the Philippines' Long Lockdowns Couldn't Contain COVID-19," *The British Medical Journal* 374 (2021): n 2063, DOI: https://doi.org/10.1136/bmj.n2063.
67 Ibid. At least one minor, a 12-year-old, died after local watchmen chased and hounded him. Another man died after police forced him to do 300 push ups when he was apprehended outside his home buying drinking water after curfew hours.
68 Michelle Ann B Eala, Ethan Angelo Maslog, Janine Patricia G. Robredo et al., "Violence Against Health-Care Workers in the Philippines," *The Lancet* 399, no. 10340 (2022): 2012–13.
69 Ibid.
70 Ibid.
71 Editorial, "COVID-19: An Ongoing Public Health Crisis in the Philippines," *The Lancet Regional Health-Western Pacific* 9 (2021): 100160.
72 Diganta Das and JJ Zhang, "Pandemic in a Smart City: Singapore's COVID-19 Management Through Technology and Society," *Urban Geography* (2020), DOI: https://doi.org/10.1080/02723638.2020.1807168.
73 Hallam Stevens and Monamie Bhadra Haines, "Trace Together: Pandemic Response, Democracy, and Technology," *East Asian Science, Technology and Society* 14, no. 3 (2020): 523–32.
74 Terence Lee and Howard Lee, "Tracing Surveillance and Auto-regulation in Singapore: 'smart' responses to COVID-19," *Media International Australia* 177, no. 1 (2020): 47–60.
75 Thomas Pepinsky, "What State-Party Relations Mean for COVID-19 Management in Southeast Asia," *Southeast Asia Insights*, January 7, 2021, https://www.brookings.edu/blog/order-from-chaos/2021/01/07/what-state-party-relations-mean-for-covid-19-management-in-southeast-asia/.
76 Chairil, "Indonesian Government's COVID-19 Measures." See also Karl Hapal, "The Philippines' COVID-19 Response: Securitising the Pandemic and Discipling the Pasaway," *Journal of Current Southeast Asian Affairs* 40, no. 2 (2021): 224–44.
77 Greg Fealy, "Jokowi in the COVID-19 era: Repressive Pluralism, Dynasticism and the Overbearing State," *Bulletin of Indonesian Economic Studies* 56, no. 3 (2020): 301–23.
78 "Human Rights Dimensions of COVID-19 Response,"*Human Rights Watch*, March 17, 2020, https://www.hrw.org/news/2020/03/19/human-rights-dimensions-covid-19-response.
79 Deepali Khanna and Nicola Nixon, "COVID-19: A Regional Response is Key for ASEAN," *The Diplomat*, December 8, 2020, https://thediplomat.com/2020/12/covid-19-a-regional-response-is-key-for-asean/.
80 Gianna Gayle Amul et al., "Responses to COVID-19 in Southeast Asia: Diverse Paths, and Ongoing Challenges," *Asian Economic Policy Review* (August 2021), doi: 10.1111/aepr.12362.
81 Michaela Grančayová, "Plagues Of Egypt – The Covid-19 Crisis And The Role Of Securitization Dilemmas in the Authoritarian Regime Survival Strategies In Egypt and Turkey," *Czech Journal Of International Relations* (2021), doi: 10.32422/mv.1766.

6 Neighbors Rally Against the Virus

The Case of SAARC

Vivek Neelakantan

South Asia—home to nearly 1.98 billion people, or a quarter of the world's population—is no stranger to either conflicts or natural disasters. Long-standing disputes between India and Pakistan or the rise of the Taliban in Afghanistan in 2021 that led to the exodus of educated women overseas underscore the political instability of the region. In April 2022, just as the coronavirus crisis was receding from Sri Lanka, the country was battling a health catastrophe: malnutrition due to the rising cost of staples, communicable diseases due to weakening preventive and curative health measures, and psychiatric disorders. The health catastrophe was an outcome of the social and political crises in the country attributed to the country's default on its external debts. Despite noticeable economic growth, South Asia has among the world's largest concentrations of poverty, illiteracy, and preventable maternal and infant mortality outside sub-Saharan Africa. The geopolitical conflict between India and Pakistan continues to undermine social spending in South Asia. For example, the decades-long confrontation of Indian and Pakistani troops along the Siachen glacier in the western Himalayas continues to cost India and Pakistan around $600 million annually, equivalent to the cost of the entire primary healthcare budget of Afghanistan between 2021 and 2023.[1]

The South Asian Association for Regional Cooperation (SAARC) is a regional grouping of South Asian Nations founded in 1985. The founding members included India, Pakistan, Bangladesh, Nepal, Bhutan, Sri Lanka, and the Maldives. For a variety of overlapping historical antecedents, the precise delimitation of South Asia as a region is not always clear, but generally incorporates the contiguous geographic boundaries extending from Afghanistan through Myanmar (Burma), including India, Pakistan, and Bangladesh.[2] At the time of the SAARC's creation, the region was undergoing political turmoil: civil wars in Sri Lanka and Afghanistan and internal security challenges for India in Punjab and in the northeastern regions. As I had examined in the introduction to the edited volume, India's locational centrality in South Asia and the asymmetry of its neighbors' size, have allowed the country to shape the contours of regional cooperation since 1947. Every state in South Asia, with the notable exception of Bhutan, has

DOI: 10.4324/9781003332060-7

had problems in bilateral relations with India in the recent past for fears of imposition of Indian hegemony. It needs to be noted here that given the geopolitical reality of SAARC with India at the helm of all bilateral disputes, SAARC was never conceived as a formal means for conflict management in South Asia.[3]

The SAARC Charter provides a clear mandate for regional cooperation. The SAARC Development Fund (established in 2010) focuses on social development. Although education and health are two key components for social development, these issues have never received enough attention at the regional level due to a paucity of funds and human resources.[4] SAARC has made limited progress in issues such as combat of terrorism, drug trafficking, or ensuring cooperation in the energy sector due to political differences between India and Pakistan.

Despite their social, linguistic, religious, political, economic, and geographic diversity, Afghanistan, Bangladesh, Bhutan, India, Maldives, Nepal, Pakistan, and Sri Lanka face common health challenges. These countries collectively bear the triple burden of communicable diseases, increasing chronic health conditions such as diabetes and hypertension, and a growing recognition of injuries, violence, and psychiatric disorders. Health systems of South Asian nations have to confront challenges such as the lack of evidence-based policies, limited health insurance and fragmentation of health services due to political and administrative decentralization. Widespread socio-economic inequities ensured that the region was a sitting duck for infectious diseases. The COVID-19 pandemic exposed the fragility of health systems across South Asia as evident in the lack of emergency response capacity, inadequate early disease warning capabilities and inadequate social support systems.

Since March 2020, the trajectory of the COVID-19 pandemic across South Asia put immense pressure on the overburdened health infrastructure of the region. Economies of the region received setbacks due to closure of businesses and loss of jobs in the informal sector. Most countries of the region, except for Pakistan, went for a hard lockdown. The pandemic provided a golden opportunity for India to revive the moribund SAARC and mend ties with its neighbors, particularly Bangladesh and Nepal. India projected itself as the "pharmacy of the world" between February 2020 and March 2021 and supplied essential medicines, ventilators, and rapid response teams consisting of medical professionals to assist countries in the immediate neighborhood. In January 2021, India supplied vaccines to other South Asian countries under the *Vaccine Maitri* (Vaccine Friendship), a humanitarian initiative based on the Sanskrit dictum of *vasudhaiva kutumbakam* (the world as one family). For example, Bangladesh was a major recipient of the COVID-19 vaccines from India under the *Vaccine Maitri* initiative.[5] The *Vaccine Maitri* initiative was in conformity with Prime Minister Narendra Modi's "Neighborhood First" doctrine that sought to disentangle India from political troubles in its immediate neighborhood and instead, compete with China for purchasing loyalties of the political elites of South Asia.

In the chapter, I argue that the COVID-19 pandemic has served not only as a catalyst but also as an inhibitor to regional integration in South Asia. India led the SAARC initiative in establishing the COVID-19 Emergency Fund. Yet, the country's political tensions with Pakistan over the revocation of the special constitutional status granted to the state of Jammu and Kashmir led to Pakistan's hesitant participation in the SAARC's response to COVID-19.

Fractured Collective Responses to COVID-19 at the National and Regional Levels

By March 11, 2020—as the number of coronavirus cases outside China increased 13-fold—the WHO officially declared COVID-19 a global pandemic. South Asia was particularly vulnerable for two reasons. First, South Asia includes half of the world's most populous cities. High urban density and rudimentary sanitation facilitate community transmission of infectious diseases. Second, public health spending in the region is among the lowest in the world, with India, Pakistan, and Bangladesh spending 3.53%, 2.9%, and 2.27% of their GDP on health, respectively.[6]

India's public health system is fragmented. There are large variations in the capacity and quality of public health service delivery across states. On the contrary, the private health sector—that provided ambulatory care to patients during the early stages of the pandemic—is largely unregulated. Health in India is a state subject. Although the eastern state of West Bengal announced in 2020 that treatment in public and private hospitals would be free for coronavirus patients, the government was unable to get large corporate private hospitals on board.[7] Likewise, the health systems in Pakistan, Afghanistan, and Bangladesh were overstretched and there were reports of doctors treating coronavirus patients without personal protective equipment. Afghanistan was particularly vulnerable to COVID-19 due to war, and an estimated 60–90% of the Afghan armed forces were possibly infected in 2020.[8] Despite these vulnerabilities, COVID-19 fatalities in South Asia were low with a case fatality rate of 1.9%, 1.3%, and 2.1% in India, Bangladesh, and Pakistan, respectively, due to poor testing rates that may have masked cases.[9] The pandemic exacerbated inequality, authoritarianism, and geopolitical rivalries across South Asia.

The World Bank warned that the lockdown-induced economic impacts could result in worsening inequality.[10] The imposition of lockdowns—intended to curb the rising infection rates across the region—led to high closure rates among business enterprises in most SAARC countries that suggest a significant loss of entrepreneurial capital and loss of informal jobs, particularly in Nepal.[11] On March 24, 2020, the Modi administration announced a nationwide lockdown across India. The lockdown was hastily announced with a four-hour notice, used little testing, and led an exodus of over 100 million inter-state and intra-state migrant workers from urban areas to the countryside. Several workers were stranded at inter-state borders and there were cases of migrants being baton-charged by the police for violating lockdown regulations. By June 2020, the central government eased regulations related to intra-state travel although not all states eased lockdown-related restrictions. The administrative fractures between the central and state governments exacerbated during the implementation of the nationwide lockdown.[12] The lockdown was particularly dire in Jammu and Kashmir after the Indian government revoked the state's special constitutional status in 2019 and suspended internet services. When the lockdown was again imposed in 2020 following COVID-19, Kashmiris were forced to rely on unstable 2 G internet connections. Consequently, local doctors struggled to download information on COVID-19.[13]

Unlike India, Pakistan did not conform to a nationwide lockdown as such a measure would lead to a deleterious impact on the informal sector. By downplaying the severity of the pandemic, the then Prime Minister Imran Khan adopted an Economy First approach that portrayed an artificial dichotomy between lives and livelihoods. Even though the first confirmed COVID-19 case in Pakistan was a pilgrim who returned from neighboring Iran (a coronavirus hotspot in March 2020), the country allowed returnees from Iran until mid-March. At the time, the Sindh provincial government, led by the opposition Pakistan People's Party, contravened Imran Khan's order and issued a lockdown order.[14] The Imran Khan administration overrode provincial lockdowns with the intervention of the Supreme Court. Pakistan's authoritarian response to the virus, such as the involvement of the military intelligence in tracing COVID-19 cases, led to the undermining of civil liberties. As the case in Pakistan, the Sri Lankan government enlisted current and ex-military generals and the central intelligence agency in the tracing of COVID cases. In Bangladesh and Nepal, journalists have been targeted for criticizing state mismanagement of the pandemic.[15]

The Maldives (with an estimated population of 541,000) recorded its first case of COVID-19 on March 7, 2020, and toward the end of March, the country recorded 18 confirmed cases and two deaths, and the first case of community transmission was recorded by mid-April 2020.[16] On April 15, 2020, the government announced a lockdown of the Greater Malé area and inter-island movements were restricted. Compliance with the Health Protection Agency's instructions related to COVID-19 prevention measures such as frequent hand-washing (72.9%), using face masks (71%), and social distancing (60%) were relatively high.[17] Border closures and the suspension of the visa-on-arrival facility adversely impacted tourism, the backbone of the Maldivian economy. The nation suffered a $450 million foreign exchange shortfall due to the economic impact of the pandemic.[18] A significant challenge facing the Maldivian government was the containment of COVID-19 among 100,000 migrant workers from other parts of South Asia—who constitute nearly 25% of the country's population—were forced to go on unpaid leave due to the closure of resorts.[19]

On March 11, 2020—when the WHO declared the novel coronavirus outbreak a pandemic—the number of coronavirus cases in South Asia were low due to limited testing. South Asian nations took individual actions, particularly testing individuals arriving from COVID-19-infected countries and their immediate contacts. Yet, it took almost 2 months for the SAARC to put aside political differences and discuss dangers posed by coronavirus. The pandemic has revealed glaring gaps in public health preparedness across the region, the lack of a robust infectious disease surveillance and control systems, and the lack of a single academic center with academic expertise to model a rapidly progressing pandemic.[20]

India shares land borders with China, Pakistan, Nepal, Bhutan, Bangladesh, and Myanmar on one hand and maritime boundaries with Maldives, Sri Lanka, Pakistan, Bangladesh, Myanmar, Thailand, and Indonesia on the other. The country's unique geopolitical location in South Asia exposes it to infectious threats that know no boundaries. Porous borders (such as the Indo-Nepal border, the Indo-Bangladesh border, the Indo-Myanmar border, or the Pakistan-Afghanistan border) require a regional response to fight pandemics. Before March 15, 2020—when Modi summoned SAARC leaders for collective action against the pandemic—confirmed COVID cases were reported in Afghanistan and Pakistan, two SAARC countries that share a long and porous border with Iran, then COVID-infected. On the contrary, no confirmed COVID-19 cases were reported in Myanmar.[21] For these reasons, India chose to reactivate the SAARC response to COVID-19 and not the BIMSTEC or The Bay of Bengal Initiative for Multi-Sectoral Technical and Economic Cooperation—a geopolitical subgrouping that includes India, Bangladesh, Myanmar, Thailand, Nepal, Bhutan, and Sri Lanka.[22]

Between 2014 and 2020, the SAARC was paralyzed due to bilateral tensions between India and Pakistan. Indo-Pak leaders have not met since 2014. The Nineteenth SAARC Summit hosted by Pakistan was boycotted by the leaders of India, Bangladesh, Bhutan, and Afghanistan due to a terrorist attack on an Indian military base in Kashmir that India blamed on Pakistani-sponsored militants. Regardless of Pakistan's attempts to derail regional consensus, Modi summoned a virtual meeting of SAARC Heads of State to chalk out a regional strategy to fight the novel coronavirus. The Indo-Pak bilateral differences were apparent in Imran Khan's decision not to attend the virtual meeting. Instead, he was represented by his Special Assistant on National Health Services, Zafar Mirza. In the meeting, Mirza proceeded to raise the controversial issue of Jammu and Kashmir that India regards as a taboo subject in bilateral and multilateral forums.[23] Likewise, in a SAARC COVID-19 follow-up virtual meeting hosted by Pakistan in April 2020, India was represented by the Director General of Health Services.[24]

On March 13, 2020, Prime Minister Narendra Modi proposed to set up the SAARC COVID-19 Emergency Fund for member states and India pledged $10 million to the fund and exhorted member states to contribute to the fund on a voluntary basis. The fund could be used by member states to meet immediate COVID-19 related expenditures. In his opening address to SAARC leaders, Modi declared:

> As we all know, COVID-19 has recently been classified by the World Health Organization as a pandemic. So far, our region has listed fewer than 150 cases. But we need to be vigilant.[25]

At the meeting, Modi offered to arrange online training capsules for disaster response teams across the region, designing software modeled on India's Integrated Disease Surveillance Portal that would help in contact tracing. Soon after the virtual meeting, the SAARC Disaster Management Center (founded in 2016) set up a website dedicated to providing an update of the COVID-19 situation in the region. The meeting delegates expressed SAARC member states' inability to fight COVID-19 alone.

India proposed that the SAARC COVID-19 Fund be implemented as a stand-alone activity outside the SAARC calendar of routine activities so that disbursement of the fund would not go through the bureaucratic grind of the SAARC Secretariat and would remain at the disposal of individual countries.[26] Apart from India, Sri Lanka pledged $5 million, Bhutan ($200,000), Bangladesh (1.5 million), Afghanistan (US $1 million), the Maldives ($100,000), and Nepal (approximately $830,000).[27] The SAARC Development Fund—established as an umbrella financial institution of the SAARC in 2005 and headquartered in Thimphu, Bhutan—committed $5 million to member states to soften the blows of financial losses and severe socio-economic impact of the pandemic.[28] On April 10, 2020, Pakistan conditionally pledged $3 million to the SAARC COVID-19 Fund.

After a few meetings, the SAARC COVID-19 fund was paralyzed due to Indo-Pak differences related to converting the fund into bilateral arrangements. Pakistan tried to score narrow political points over India by tying its COVID-19 Emergency Fund to the SAARC Secretariat. Pakistan contended that its COVID-19 contribution should be finalized through consultations with SAARC member states in accordance with Article 10 of the SAARC Charter.[29]

On the contrary, India was unequivocal that the Emergency Response Fund was not a traditional fund as there was no central administrator, no central pooling of money, and no central administrator who would monitor the use of funds by the recipient country. India asserted that when SAARC member states pledged a certain amount, they would keep the fund separate at their disposal for use of other countries of the regional grouping. Requests for using the fund would have to be sent individually by recipient nations to the donor state within the SAARC grouping.[30] Furthermore, when Modi tweeted on March 13, 2020, "I would like to propose that the leadership of SAARC nations chalk out a strong strategy to fight coronavirus," there were eyebrows raised in South Asian capitals about India's possible domination of the SAARC as the regional grouping had not exactly figured in Modi's foreign policy between 2016 and 2019.[31]

The Geopolitics of the COVID-19 Vaccine in South Asia: The Case of India's *Vaccine Maitri*

The COVID-19 vaccine is regarded as a new tool of health diplomacy. China and India (and to a lesser extent Russia and the US) compete to project their geopolitical influence in South Asia through donations or inking of vaccine purchase agreements with countries that have limited access to vaccines. Since the coronavirus outbreak in Wuhan (2019), China has been on a diplomatic rollercoaster, garnering international sympathy as well as accusations from the US for cover-up of the initial outbreak. In April 2020, after a successful mitigation of the pandemic at home, the Chinese government launched a public relations campaign that branded the country as a global health leader under the "Health Silk Road" moniker.[32] The Chinese conceptualized COVID-19 vaccine diplomacy as a bilateral construct outside the WHO-led COVAX consortium.[33] On the contrary, India has not only pledged COVID-19 vaccines to the COVAX consortium but is also using vaccine diplomacy to mend troubled relationships with its immediate neighbors such as Bangladesh and Nepal through bilateral means rather than the SAARC.

There is a lack of consensus among South Asian scholars about the nature of India's vaccine diplomacy. Smruti Pattanaik notes that India's health diplomacy enhanced its soft power projection and helped to project an image of the country that was concerned about its neighbors.[34] On the contrary, scholars such as Ambar Basu and Parameswari Mukherjee contend that India launched the *Vaccine Maitri* program on January 21, 2021, purported to extend a neighborly hand to a select few developmentally poorer South Asian countries so that they would not be left behind in their fight against COVID-19. Although India's gesture was advertised as an act of friendship, the campaign was aimed to advance India's burgeoning goals of developmental expansion in South Asia.[35] The vaccines produced domestically are not only expected to cover the people of India but also those of neighboring states. India would not only be *atma nirbhar* (self-reliant), according to Modi, but also look out to save humanity.[36] The *atma nirbhar* trope of Modi is noteworthy as *Atma Nirbhar Bharat* (India) would create pathways for increased flow of global capital into the country and accord a prominent role for the country's science and technology in the global chain.[37]

Critics of *Vaccine Maitri* have pointed out that Modi's vision of *atma nirbhar Bharat* in vaccine production is intricately tied to the paradigm of development and its alignment with a neo-liberal movement which calls for a capital-led transformation of developing countries.[38] Such a transformation implies acquiring a capacity to provide sufficiently for the country's citizens and being able to reach a point of surplus that might be used to save citizens of development-wise-less-fortunate nations.[39] In India's case the goal was to "save" citizens of neighboring countries by deploying the country's homegrown vaccines: Covaxin and Covishield. In turn, India's capital networks would gain access to natural resources and consumer resources of neighboring countries. Likewise, China has supplied vaccines to Nepal, Bangladesh, and Sri Lanka, first as grants, then commercially. China wants India to acquiesce itself to the idea that the former is a leading power in South Asia. To this end, China has befriended India's neighbors on the basis of "Five Principles of Peaceful Co-Existence" to eventually persuade India to accept the idea that New Delhi and Beijing can peacefully co-exist in South Asia.[40] The "Five Principles of Peaceful Co-Existence" are linked to the Chinese cultural principle of *Tianxia* (All Under Heaven) that has influenced the China's policy towards India's neighbors.[41] China has increased economic engagement with South Asia and has oriented its vaccine diplomacy to provide a counterweight to Indian influence in the region.

Bangladesh received the top priority under India's *Vaccine Maitri* program. Since 2020, India's public image in Bangladesh suffered a downturn. First, India announced the controversial Citizenship Amendment Act which grants citizenship to persecuted non-Muslims from Pakistan, Bangladesh, and Afghanistan. Second, the Indian government introduced the National Register of Citizens to identify illegal Bangladeshi immigrants in the northeastern state of Assam. China derived strategic advantage from the situation with its state-run firms landing big infrastructure projects, outbidding Indian companies in Bangladesh. In August 2020, although Bangladesh permitted Chinese private company Sinovac Biotech to stage clinical trials of the coronavirus vaccine, there was controversy over the financial resource contribution.[42] Bangladesh's close ties with China and India gave it leverage to ensure that both countries supply a large quantity of the vaccine at low prices. In January 2021, India gifted 3.3 million doses of the Covishield vaccine—manufactured by the Serum Institute of India, a private company—followed by 7 million vaccine doses purchased by Bangladesh from the same company.[43] However, soon after the outbreak of the second wave of the pandemic in India in April 2021, the country suspended vaccine exports to its neighborhood. Bangladesh was left with limited choices except to approach China.

Beijing has been cultivating close ties with Dhaka to secure a foothold in the Bay of Bengal region and leverage its Belt and Road initiative.[44] Chinese vaccine manufacturer Sinopharm gifted 500,000 doses of the vaccine to Bangladesh on May 12, 2021.[45] The gift was preceded by a warning by China's ambassador to Bangladesh Li Jimming that Sino-Bangladeshi ties would be damaged if Bangladesh joined the Quad alliance that China terms as an anti-Beijing Club.[46] Incidentally, India is a member of the alliance.

In April 2020, the Chinese Defense Minister, Wei Fenghe visited Bangladesh and called for enhanced military cooperation between the two countries to prevent the Quad alliance from setting up a military alliance in South Asia. Such warnings from China carry a coercive undertone to vaccine diplomacy in Bangladesh.

As a small but populous developing country—that shares a maritime and land border with India and in close proximity to China—Bangladesh is challenged with the task of maintaining meaningful partnerships with India and China while safeguarding its sovereignty. The country sought to minimize its dependence on India and China and instead, authorized the emergency use of the Russian Sputnik V vaccine in April 2021. But as the arrival of the Russian vaccine doses were delayed, Bangladesh decided to source approximately 4.55 million doses of COVID-19 vaccine donated by Japan through the COVAX facility, between July and December 2021.[47]

As the case in Bangladesh, *Vaccine Maitri* provided an opportunity for India to recalibrate its bilateral relations with Nepal. The bilateral relations hit a downturn in 2019 following the Kalapani territorial dispute—an area situated at the strategic China-India-Nepal trijunction.[48] Nepal began its vaccination drive on January 27, 2021, with 1.1 million doses of the Covishield vaccine supplied by the Serum Institute of India on grant-assistance basis. Furthermore, the country purchased 1 million doses of the vaccine from the Institute and received 0.34 million doses of Covishield from the COVAX consortium.[49]

During the unforeseen second wave of COVID-19 in Nepal, there was an 88.8% rise in new cases between April 5 and April 11, 2021.[50] At the same time, India had imposed a moratorium on export of vaccine doses to neighboring countries as the country itself was battling the second wave. Not surprisingly, Nepal's nationwide vaccination drive was suspended. By mid-2021, only 2% of the country's population was adequately vaccinated.[51] The country tilted closer to China in May 2021 to roll out COVID-19 related requirements for its population amidst the upcoming national elections. Nepal has chosen balancing between India and China whereas Bhutan has chosen to bandwagon with India. Nepal and Bhutan are both landlocked mountainous states sandwiched between China and India. Yet, their policies have followed very different trajectories.[52]

India's *Vaccine Maitri* was partially successful in Bhutan. Aided in its efforts by *Vaccine Maitri*, the country managed to vaccinate nearly 94% of its adult population with the first dose by March 2021.[53] As of 2020, the country had only 37 doctors serving a population of approximately 720,000.[54] Despite logistical challenges, factors contributing to the relative success of Bhutan in managing COVID-19 between 2020 and 2021 included the country's robust healthcare system. Being a signatory to the Alma Ata Declaration on Primary Healthcare (1978), the country has expanded its primary health network to cover 95% of the population. By 1991, the country achieved Universal Child Immunization.[55] The success of the nationwide COVID-19 vaccination program was in no small measure due to the government's enlistment of the Zhung Dratsang or the Buddhist clergy in determining the auspicious time of vaccination, a strategy that enabled the Ministry of Health adequate time to organize the campaign's logistics.[56] *Desuups* or volunteers appointed by the king delivered vaccines to health centers and educated the Bhutanese about COVID control measures.

India recorded more than 300,000 coronavirus cases daily during the peak of the second wave and suffered from an acute scarcity of medical oxygen and beds. Bhutan assisted India with the supply of medical oxygen. With India's second wave of COVID-19 peaking between April and May 2021, the country suspended vaccine exports to Bhutan. With no vaccines in sight and the looming deadline for administering the second dose to the population, Bhutan was forced to look for alternative COVID-19 vaccine sources. By May 2021, there was a 66.2% increase in daily coronavirus cases in Bhutan—particularly in the districts of Phuentsholing, Samdurp, and Trashigang—bordering India.[57] The country was open to all options related to vaccine procurement, including mixing and matching or heterologous inoculation that involved using a different second vaccine.[58] By July 2021, the US pledged around 500,000 Moderna vaccine doses to the country through the global COVAX consortium. Additionally, China sent a consignment of 50,000 Sinopharm doses to Bhutan when India repurposed its vaccine supplies to meet domestic requirements.

China does not maintain formal diplomatic relations with Bhutan. Yet, China's dispatch of the Sinopharm vaccine to Bhutan should be placed within the context of the former's inauguration of the China-South Asian Countries Poverty Alleviation and Development Center and the China-South Asia Emergency Reserve Center. The China-South Asia Emergency Reserve Center is intended to assist the region to tackle the COVID pandemic and other disasters.[59] Both centers are parts of China's efforts to foster long-term cooperation with South Asian nations under the Belt and Road Initiative, seen within Indian foreign policy circles as an effort to undermine SAARC.

Sri Lanka—strategically straddling the Indian Ocean submarine data cable routes—has emerged as a major theater of vaccine diplomacy. Major vaccine producing nations, particularly India, China, the US, and Russia are keen to gain a strategic foothold in the island nation. Sri Lanka launched its nationwide vaccination campaign on January 29, 2021, following the delivery of 500,000 doses of the Covishield vaccine by India as a gift under the *Vaccine Maitri* followed by an additional purchase of 500,000 vaccines. But India could not fulfill its commitment to supply vaccine doses to Sri Lanka by April 2021 due to the outbreak of the second wave and the island nation had to diversify its sources of vaccine supplies.

Apart from India, China sanctioned a $500 million loan to Sri Lanka to offset the setbacks suffered by the latter due to the COVID-19 pandemic.

Australia pledged AU $5.5 million to assist Sri Lanka with its COVID-19 response; Japan granted $16.2 million; and the US $8 million.[60] On May 14, 2021, the World Bank loaned Sri Lanka $80.5 million for organizing the logistics of the campaign whereas the Asian Development Bank loaned $150 million to the island nation for the procurement of COVID-19 vaccines.[61] Additionally, the Serum Institute of India pledged 264,000 doses of Covishield through the COVAX consortium; the US donated over 100,000 doses of Pfizer-BioNTech COVID-19 vaccines under the COVAX consortium; and China donated 1.4 million doses of Sinopharm.[62] The island nation exceeded the expectations of the WHO as it succeeded in fully vaccinating 53.3% of its population by September 2021.[63] Yet, Sri Lanka's vaccination program was overshadowed by controversy.

In the nationwide vaccination campaign, the government prioritized the vaccination of children. The Pfizer vaccine was marketed in the local Sri Lankan media as the "most desirable vaccine."[64] A report from *The Colombo Telegraph*, an online Sri Lankan newspaper run by exiled journalists, expressed concern about the authorization of the Pfizer vaccine for Emergency Use in the island nation. The author of the report expressed concern about the safety and efficacy of the Pfizer vaccine, "Questions now arise as to whether Sri Lanka children are being rendered 'guinea pigs' for Big Pharmaceutical companies and their vaccines authorized for Emergency Use only, which were developed at 'warped speed' in less than a year, and untested in Asian countries?"[65]

Apart from safety and efficacy concerns, skepticism toward the Pfizer vaccine in the island nation could be attributed to the acrimonious relationship between the State Pharmaceutical Corporation (SPC) and Pfizer, dating back to the 1970s. Under the leadership of Sri Lankan Pharmacist Senaka Bibile, the SPC began a centralized procurement of a rationalized list of finished drugs; the purchase of intermediate chemicals for local manufacture of pharmaceuticals; non-observance of patents; and a change from brand to generic names.[66] Transnational pharmaceutical companies—finding their oligopolistic pricing and profits cut—launched an insidious campaign against low-cost local suppliers.

Sri Lanka was unable to leverage vaccine diplomacy to meet its domestic requirements. There were allegations that the island nation had paid a higher price for the Sinopharm vaccine than either Bangladesh or Nepal.[67]

As a small island nation, the Maldives does not have many foreign policy options other than align with either India or China. To serve its national interests, the Maldives— like many other small countries, particularly Nepal— entered into what Alyson Bailes, Bradley Thayer, and Baldur Thorhallson term as the concept of "alliance of shelter."[68] During the presidency of Abdulla Yameen (2013–18), the Maldives agreed to join China's Belt and Road Initiative, Chinese companies invested in civic infrastructure projects of the island nation and were accused of pushing the country into indebtedness.[69]

In 2018, Ibrahim Solih won the presidential election following his criticism of Chinese infrastructural projects in the Maldives. The Solih administration followed an "India First" policy. "India First" seeks to reconcile India's growing presence in the Maldives against the fierce tradition of Maldivian independence.[70] Solih's first official visit in December 2018 was to India. During Solih's meeting with Modi, the latter announced a $1.4 billion loan to the Maldives to enable the indebted nation repay its loans to China.[71]

For India, vaccine diplomacy in the Maldives has given it a rejoinder to China, after years of watching Beijing's inroads in South Asia and the Indian Ocean region. China offered infrastructure projects and loans that India struggled to match due to a layered bureaucracy and a general economic slowdown after 2016. Due to the geopolitical rivalry between China and India, the Maldives managed to get vaccine doses from both. On January 20, 2021, India donated 100,000 doses of Covishield to Malé and an additional 100,000 doses were received by February when the country commenced its vaccination drive, officially known as *COVID-19 Dhifaau* (COVID-19 Defense).[72] Following a request from the Solih administration, Bangladesh dispatched a team of 23 healthcare professionals to assist in the nationwide vaccination program. The enlistment of Bangladeshi healthcare professionals in the national vaccination campaign was intended to overcome linguistic barriers and make the COVID-19 vaccine acceptable to migrant workers, a majority of whom hailed from Bangladesh. Making the vaccine free and accessible to citizens and migrant workers alike was a salient feature of the Maldivian government's COVID-19 response. The beginnings of *Covid-19 Dhifaau* seemed promising as nearly 60% of the country's population received at least the first dose of the vaccine.[73]

The Maldives was initially using Covishield from India, Pfizer, and Sinopharm in its nationwide vaccination campaign. By May 2021—with the outbreak of the second wave of COVID-19 in India, fueled by the deadly Delta variant—the *Vaccine Maitri* program was suspended and the Soli government had to approach Russia for the Sputnik V vaccine. Between January 20 and July 6, 2021, as a third wave of COVID-19 swept through the Maldives, the number of COVID-positive cases grew exponentially from 14,712 to 74,585.[74] The third COVID-19 wave affected the pace of vaccination due to the continuation of enhanced mobility restrictions. Nevertheless, the country managed to vaccinate 65.6% of the population with two doses of the vaccine.[75] As India was affected by the second wave, the Maldives turned to Russia to redress shortage of vaccine doses.

Unlike the rest of South Asia, Pakistan was not a direct beneficiary of India's *Vaccine Maitri*. The Indian Ministry of External Affairs did not receive requests for vaccine from Pakistan.[76] Nevertheless, the country received Indian-made vaccines through the COVAX consortium although supplies were delayed as India decided to divert all supplies for domestic use, following the onset of the second COVID wave in April 2021.[77] Pakistan was forced to reengineer its vaccination strategy and approach China and

Russia for vaccine supplies. Pakistan did offer to send relief material to India during the second wave but exhorted India to release Kashmiri political prisoners.[78] The *Vaccine Maitri* could have revitalized Indo-Pak bilateral relations that reached a new nadir following terrorist attacks on an Indian military base in Kashmir in 2016 and contain rising Chinese influence in Pakistan.

Afghanistan is of geopolitical significance to both Pakistan and India due to its proximity to the hydrocarbon rich Central Asian republics. The country has shown interest in multilateral energy pipelines connecting Turkmenistan, Afghanistan, Pakistan, and India which could bring in much-needed transit revenue and reflects the country's policy that seeks balanced relations with India and Pakistan.[79] For China, stability in Afghanistan is a necessary prerequisite for the success of the China-Pakistan Economic Corridor, a Belt and Road initiative that seeks to improve connectivity between China and Central Asia through Afghanistan. Given the strategic significance of Afghanistan for India's connectivity to Central Asia, the former was a beneficiary of *Vaccine Maitri* and received 500,000 doses of Covishield by February 7, 2021 and 468,000 vaccine doses in March through the COVAX.[80] Due to the onset of the second COVID-19 wave in India, Afghanistan's fledgling vaccination program was interrupted.

Vaccine skepticism is common in Afghanistan where few residents follow pandemic-related protocols. Skeptics point to government statistics that reveal 2800 COVID-19 deaths in a country of over 38 million people.[81] Other skeptics contend that if the vaccine were effective, India would not have entered the second wave.[82] Conspiracy theories in Afghan society range from the vaccines being a Central Intelligence Agency (CIA) project to track and target Afghans to a widespread but mistaken belief that that the COVID-19 vaccine is made with ingredients proscribed by Islam.[83] The claims of CIA interference in using the COVID-19 vaccine in tracking and targeting Afghans have a precedent dating back to 2011. At the time, Shikal Afridi—a physician working with the CIA—used the Hepatitis-B vaccination campaign as a pretext to track the whereabouts of Osama bin Laden, the founder of the pan-Islamic militant group al-Qaeda, that led to his killing.[84] As a result of vaccine skepticism and hesitancy, less than 3% of Afghans were vaccinated.[85]

Having analyzed the implementation of India's *Vaccine Maitri* initiative, it would be inevitable to conclude that official pronouncements of India's role in addressing the global demand for vaccines as a demonstration of *Atma Nirbhar Bharat* should be read as attempts to portray Indian exceptionalism. Furthermore, the Government of India portrays the *Vaccine Maitri* initiative as a government initiative to combat vaccine nationalism. But the bulk of vaccine exports overseas by the Serum Institute of India were fulfilled as a part of its contractual obligations to its collaborators Astra Zeneca and COVAX. It is creditable that India donated vaccines to South Asian neighbors and Myanmar unlike the US that was sitting on unused stocks of Astra Zeneca vaccines but reluctant to share them with developing countries.[86] Yet, one could argue that India's vaccine donations to South Asian neighbors and Myanmar were driven by geopolitical calculations such as the need to check Chinese influence. Furthermore, clubbing India's vaccine donations with commercial sales by private companies such as the Serum Institute of India and Bharat Biotech (the manufacturer of Covaxin) creates a false impression that the Indian government was a major vaccine supplier.

During the second wave of the pandemic—with the expansion of the nationwide vaccination program and a public backlash when it became known that more vaccine doses had been exported than used domestically—the Modi administration was forced to impose a moratorium on vaccine exports.[87] Consequently, the Serum Institute also had to halt its overseas shipments and reneged on agreements with Astra Zeneca although the former had committed to meet the latter's global vaccine supply. The Indian government categorically denied that there was any moratorium on vaccine exports overseas even though it prevented exports. For example, the delay of Indian vaccine shipments to Nepal and Bangladesh by May 2021 led to delays in administering second vaccine doses. The second wave of the pandemic in India opened the door for China to export vaccines to both countries. If India had aspired to be the pharmacy of the world, the government's abrupt reversal of vaccine exports—that coincided with the outbreak of the second wave of the pandemic—was likely to have damaged the country's reputation as the "first responder" to regional crises.

Conclusion: Why Does a Regional Approach to COVID-19 Matter in South Asia?

Since 2004, India's humanitarian assistance is largely directed to its neighborhood. Under the guise of "first responder," India is signaling its global aspirations to be a leading regional actor in responding to emergencies in its neighborhood. As India's Minister for External Affairs and Former Foreign Secretary S. Jaishankar put it, "India's foreign policy dimension is to aspire to be a leading power, rather than just a balancing power…(and) a willingness to shoulder greater global responsibilities."[88] India's aspirations as a leading power are related to the country's enhanced economic and military capabilities. For instance, India has contributed to infrastructure projects in Bangladesh, invested in hydropower projects in Nepal and Bhutan, and has assisted post-civil war reconstruction in Sri Lanka. India's insistence on emphasizing territorial sovereignty in its humanitarian assistance narrative results in bilateral aid to its South Asian neighbor while the country's contribution to multilateral organizations such as SAARC or BIMSTEC have been less significant. Hostile Indo-Pak bilateral relations are partly to blame for India circumventing the mechanism of the SAARC Secretariat and instead, respond to emergencies in neighboring South Asian nations on a bilateral basis.

The 2004 Indian Ocean Tsunami provided an impetus for the establishment of the SAARC Disaster Management Center although no SAARC-level contingent has ever been deployed to member states to assist in the management of emergencies. During the early stages of the COVID-19 pandemic across South Asia, India proposed the SAARC COVID-19 Emergency Fund and pledged $10 million for coordinating emergency relief. Although the Fund sparked initial enthusiasm of SAARC member states—with all countries agreeing to contribute—most aid was carried out on a bilateral basis. In short, as the Fund is not operationalized through the SAARC Secretariat, it is seen as another Indian-led initiative.

In 2021, South Asia drove the global surge in COVID-19. The region accounts for 33.4% of the world's poor who have suffered from economic disruptions due to lockdowns between 2020 and 2021. Early responses to COVID-19 across the region were incoherent. India and Bangladesh elected for a nationwide lockdown that was subsequently followed by massive efforts to scale up social security. On the contrary, Pakistan instituted a program of Emergency Cash Transfers to cushion the poor from the economic shock of the pandemic.[89] An early and free exchange of ideas and options across the region could have led to much more coherent policy response and mutual learnings of SAARC member states that would benefit of those on low incomes. During the pandemic, regional cooperation was limited to setting up of the token SAARC COVID-19 Emergency Fund whereas there was negligible collaboration on COVID surveillance or early warning of risks from variants. The capacity of South Asia to mount an emergency response to COVID-19 was partly contingent on national and regional diagnostic capabilities and securing medical supplies. Whereas India scaled up its COVID-19 testing and built-up capacity for the production of personal protective equipment and oximeters, other South Asian nations spent a fortune importing medical supplies from overseas that could have otherwise been sourced from within the region at a fraction of the cost.

The global program to develop safe and effective coronavirus vaccines has yielded results due to Operation Warp Speed—a public-private partnership initiated by the US government in May 2020— that accelerated the development, manufacturing, and distribution of COVID-19 vaccines. The project involved pulling in contract manufacturers from the US and Europe and it required creating complex supply chains to import raw materials. Some pharmaceutical companies such as Astra Zeneca have engaged global contract manufacturers such as the Serum Institute of India in emerging economies to meet the ever-growing global demand for the COVID-19 vaccine. Furthermore, the competitive procurement of vaccines by the US and other high-income countries has fed the widespread assumption of vaccine nationalism that each country would be solely responsible for its own population.[90] Wealthy nations such as Australia, Japan, and Canada— that accounted for 1% of the global coronavirus cases in 2021—locked up more doses than Latin America and the Caribbean, a region with more than 17% of the world's COVID cases.[91] An uncoordinated patchwork of immunity globally could facilitate the development of mutant coronavirus strains that could alter the effectiveness of vaccines. Vaccine Nationalism can be countered if South Asia acts as a bloc.

India has widely been regarded as the "Pharmacy Capital of the World," without taking into account the manufacturing capacities of its South Asian neighbors. Augmentation of vaccine production in itself is not sufficient to remedy shortages in parts of South Asia. There is a need to agree on shared technology ownership/transfer and an equity-based regional distribution model based on priority groups defined based on assessment of risks and vulnerabilities.[92] Securing equitable access to COVID-19 vaccines remains a collective challenge to South Asian nations that need to act as a bloc to request vaccines from high-income countries using a combination of collective needs assessment and diplomacy.

A regional approach to the COVID-19 pandemic is critical for reinventing global health mechanisms such as the COVAX. Equity, the cardinal principle guiding COVAX, is distorted by developed countries that have purchased vaccine stocks directly from vaccine manufacturers and developed stockpiles. The shortcomings of COVAX are twofold. First, in the setting of vaccine scarcity, in which suppliers are unable to deliver doses as scheduled and countries are banning exports to keep vaccines at home, there is a risk that COVAX aid-recipient states will fall further down the priority list, awaiting the leftover vaccines from the rich country stockpiles.[93] Second, COVAX is used by developed countries and pharmaceutical companies to overlook demands for patent waivers.[94] COVAX has become a smokescreen for an inequitable global health system. As such, the emphasis on a donor-based model of vaccine aid distracts leaders from the ideologies, economic systems, and patent regimes, which leaves vaccine distribution to the caprices of the market rather than global health priorities.

The SAARC has a major role to play in transforming COVAX from a neo-colonial purchase-donate model to a model that facilitates domestic capacity building across South Asia related to the production of COVID-19 vaccine. As Shashika Bandara, Soumyadeep Bhoumik, Veena Sriram et al. contend, "Access to vaccines or essential medicines, a vital component of the right to health, should not be dependent on charitable inclinations, economic or political interests of HICs [High Income Countries], or private corporations—a regional effort is required to change the status quo."[95]

Notes

1 Zulfiqar A. Bhutta, Arun Mitra, Afsah Salman et al., "Conflict, Extremism, Resilience and Peace in South Asia: Can Covid-19 Provide a Bridge for Peace and Rapprochement?", *The British Medical Journal (BMJ)* 375 (2021): e 067384, DOI: http://dx.doi.org/10.1136/BMJ-2021-067384.

2 Lawrence Saez, *The South Asian Association for Regional Cooperation: An Emerging Collaboration Architecture* (Abingdon, Oxon: Routledge, 2011).

3 Rajshree Jetly, "Conflict Management Strategies in ASEAN: Perspectives for SAARC," *The Pacific Review* 16, no. 1 (2003): 53–76.

4 Zahid Shahab Ahmed and Munir Hussain, "South Asian Regionalism, Social Development and COVID-19: Lessons for SAARC from the EU's Social Model," *Asian Journal of Comparative Politics* (2022), DOI: 10.1177/20578911221104275.

5 Of the nine million doses of Indian vaccine dispatched to Bangladesh between January and March 2021, seven million doses were commercial purchases whereas two million were grant assistance from the Indian government. Refer A. J. Vinayak, "Vaccine Maitri: Sanjeevani for the World," *The Hindu Businessline*, March 4, 2021, https://www.thehindubusinessline.com/news/variety/vaccine-maitri-a-sanjeevini-for-the-world/article62178717.ece.

6 Rupert Stone, "COVID-19 in South Asia: Mirror and Catalyst," *Asian Affairs* 51, no. 3 (2020): 542–68.

7 Kamala Thiagarajan, "COVID-19 Exposes the High Cost of Reliance on India's Private Healthcare," *BMJ* 370 (2020): m 3506, DOI: 10.1136/bmj.m3506.

8 Stone, "COVID-19 in South Asia," 545.

9 Ibid., 546.

10 The World Bank, *COVID-19 in South Asia: An Unequal Shock, An Uncertain Recovery* (Washington, DC: World Bank, 2022).

11 Ibid.

12 For details related to the first wave of COVID-19 across India, see Marcos Cueto, Vivek Neelakantan and Gabriel Lopes, "The Regulation of Necropolitics: Governmental Responses to COVID-19 in Brazil and India in the First Year of the Pandemic," *SCIELO Preprints* (June 2022), https://doi.org/10.1590/SciELOPreprints.4244.

13 Stone, "COVID-19 in South Asia," 555.

14 Ibid., 553.

15 Ibid., 555.

16 Sheena Moosa, Mariyam Suzana, Fazeel Najeeb et al., *Preliminary Report: Study on Socio-Economic Aspects of Covid-19 in the Maldives, Round Two*, June 2020 (Malé: The Maldives National University and Health Protection Agency, 2020).

17 Ibid.

18 Samantha Mallempati, "The Virus and Island States: How Sri Lanka and the Maldives Cope with COVID-19," *Indian Council of World Affairs*, April 3, 2020, https://icwa.in/show_content.php?lang=1&level=3&ls_id=4672&lid=3515.

19 Ibid.

20 Zulfiqar A. Bhutta, Buddha Basnyat, Samir Saha and Ramanan Laxminarayan, Editorial "Covid-19 Risks and Response in South Asia," *BMJ* 368 (2020): m1190, DOI: https://doi.org/10.1136/bmj.m1190.

21 K. Yhome, "COVID-19 and SAARC Diplomacy," *Observer Research Foundation Health Express*, March 23, 2020, https://www.orfonline.org/expert-speak/covid-19-crisis-and-saarc-diplomacy-63598/.

22 Ibid.

23 Pradeep Taneja and Azad Singh Bali, "India's Domestic and Foreign Policy Responses to COVID-19," *The Round Table: The Commonwealth Journal of International Affairs* 110, no. 1 (2021): 46–61.

24 "India's Participation in the Video Conference of SAARC Leaders on COVID-19 Hosted by Pakistan," *Government of India Ministry of External Affairs Media Center*, April 23, 2020, https://mea.gov.in/press-releases.htm?dtl/32649/Indias_participation_in_the_video_conference_of_SAARC_Health_Ministers_on_COVID19_hosted_by_Pakistan.

25 "Coronavirus: Modi Proposes SAARC COVID-19 Emergency Fund for SAARC Nations: Offers \$10 Million," *Scroll.in*, March 15, 2020, https://scroll.in/latest/956263/coronavirus-modi-proposes-covid-19-emergency-fund-for-saarc-nations-offers-10-million.

26 Smruti Pattanaik, Commentary "SAARC COVID-19 Fund: Calibrating a Regional Response to the Pandemic," *Strategic Analysis* 44, no. 3 (2020): 241–52.

27 "Coronavirus Disease (COVID-19): SAARC Region," *SAARC Disaster Management Centre*, http://www.covid19-sdmc.org/.

28 Nazia Hussain, "Impetus for SAARC Revival," *RSIS Commentary* 76 (April 24, 2020), https://www.rsis.edu.sg/wp-content/uploads/2020/04/CO20076.pdf.

29 SAARC, "SAARC Charter," https://www.saarc-sec.org/index.php/about-saarc/saarc-charter. Article 10 of the SAARC Charter stipulates that decisions at all levels shall be taken on the basis of unanimity.

30 "SAARC COVID-19 Response Fund: After Pak's Demand, India Rules Out Secretariat's Role," *The Wire*, April 10, 2020, https://thewire.in/south-asia/saarc-covid-19-emergency-response-fund-pakistan-india-secretariat.

31 "Pakistan Joins Neighbours in Welcoming Modi's Call for SAARC to Combat COVID-19," *The Wire*, March 14, 2020, https://thewire.in/south-asia/saarc-modi-pakistan-coronavirus.

32 Seow Ting Lee, "Vaccine Diplomacy: Nation Branding and China's Soft Power Play," *Place Branding and Public Diplomacy* (2021), DOI: https://doi.org/10.1057/s41254-021-00224-4.

33 The COVAX or COVID-19 Vaccines Global Access is a global initiative aimed at the equitable distribution of COVID-19 vaccines, led by the WHO, GAVI vaccine alliance and Coalition for Epidemic Preparedness Innovations. Depending on how much they have paid in, rich countries can access vaccine doses for 10–50% of their population whereas poorer countries can access vaccine doses for 20%. The COVAX's unique selling mechanism is that every nation in the world can get the COVID-19 vaccine regardless of purchasing power.

34 See for e.g., Smruti Patttanaik, "COVID-19 AND India's Regional Diplomacy," *South Asian Survey* 28, no. 1 (2021): 92–110.

35 Ambar Basu and Parameswari Mukherjee, "India's COVID Gestures: From *Maitri* to Coloniality," *Communication and/Critical Cultural Studies* 19, no. 2 (2022): 134–39.

36 Basu and Mukherjee, "India's COVID Gestures," 136.

37 Ibid.

38 Ibid.

39 Ibid.

40 Anuttama Banerji, "India's Flawed Vaccine Diplomacy," *Stimson South Asian Voices Project*, June 25, 2021, https://www.stimson.org/2021/indias-flawed-vaccine-diplomacy/#.

41 Ibid.

42 Khanindra Ch. Das, "Financial Interdependence Since COVID-19: China and South Asia," *China Report* 58, no. 2 (2022): 131–51.

43 Sohini Bose, "Bangladesh: Navigating Diplomacy Challenges in Search for Vaccines," in *The Dynamics of Vaccine Diplomacy in India's Neighbourhood*, Sohini Bose edited (New Delhi: Observer Research Foundation Report No. 145, 2021), https://www.orfonline.org/research/the-dynamics-of-vaccine-diplomacy-in-indias-neighbourhood/.

44 The Belt and Road Initiative, a global infrastructure strategy, was introduced by Chinese President Xi Jinping in 2013. It is considered the centerpiece of China's foreign policy. The Initiative is an important Chinese attempt to

sustain its economic growth by exploring new forms of international cooperation in Asia, Europe and Africa and assert greater international influence
by drawing from the country's experiences. For details see Yiping Huang,
"Understanding China's Belt & Road Initiative: Motivation, Framework and
Assessment," *China Economic Review* 40 (2016): 314–21.

45 Bose, "Bangladesh Navigating Diplomacy Challenges."
46 Ibid. The Quad is a geopolitical grouping that includes India, Japan, Australia and the US, aimed at maintaining a rules-based order and a free, inclusive and open Indo-Pacific.
47 Press Releases "The Provision of COVID-19 Vaccines to the People's
Republic of Bangladesh through the COVAX Facility," Ministry of Foreign
Affairs of Japan, December 13, 2021, https://www.mofa.go.jp/press/release/
press6e_000356.html.
48 In November 2019, the Indian Home Ministry issued a new edition of the
Indian political map that depicted the disputed Kalapani region in the
Greater Himalayas as within India's borders. The Nepalese government
immediately issued objection to the map as it identifies the region as an unset-
tled territory as part of the country's Sudurpaschim province. For details
related to the Kalapani dispute refer Sohini Nayak, "India and Nepal's Kalapani Border Dispute: An Explainer," *ORF Brief* 356 (April 2020), https://www.
orfonline.org/wp-content/uploads/2020/04/ORF_IssueBrief_356_India-Nepal-
Kalapani.pdf.
49 Sohini Nayak, "Nepal and Bhutan: Mountains of Challenges in the Hima-
layan States," in *The Dynamics of Vaccine Diplomacy in India's Neighbourhood*, Sohini Bose edited (New Delhi: Observer Research Foundation
Report No. 145, 2021), https://www.orfonline.org/research/the-dynamics-
of-vaccine-diplomacy-in-indias-neighbourhood/.
50 Ibid.
51 Ibid.
52 See also Nitasha Kaul, "Beyond India and China: Bhutan as a Small State in
International Relations," *International Relations of the Asia-Pacific* 22, no. 2
(2022): 297–337.
53 Thinley Dorji and Saran Tenzin Tamang, Commentary "Bhutan's Experience
with COVID-19 Vaccine in 2021," *BMJ* 6 (2021): e 005977, DOI: https://doi.
org/10.1136%2Fbmjgh-2021-005977.
54 Paulina Villegas, "Bhutan Fully Vaccinates 90 Percent of Eligible Adults Within
a Week," *The Washington Post*, July 28, 2021, https://www.washingtonpost.
com/world/2021/07/28/bhutan-covid-vaccination/.
55 Ibid.
56 Ian Christopher N. Rocha, Letter to the Editor "Employing Medical
Anthropology Approach as an Additional Public Health Strategy in Promoting COVID-19 Vaccine Acceptance in Bhutan," *The International Journal of Health Planning and Management* (2021), DOI: https://doi.org/10.1002/
hpm.3191.
57 Sohini Nayak, "Nepal and Bhutan."
58 Suhasini Haidar, "Hit By India's Vaccine Export Ban, Bhutan Seeks
Help," *The Hindu*, June 27, 2021, https://www.thehindu.com/news/
international/hit-by-indias-vaccine-export-ban-bhutan-seeks-help/
article35006213.ece.
59 Elizabeth Roche, "China Sends 50,000 Doses of Sinopharm Covid Vaccines to Bhutan," *Mint*, July 15, 2021, https://www.livemint.com/news/
world/china-sends-50-000-doses-of-sinopharm-covid-vaccines-to-
bhutan-11626337840042.html.

60 Mahnoor Hayat, Mohammad Uzair, Rafay Ali Syed,Muhammad Arshad and Shahid Bashir, "Status of COVID-19 Vaccination Around South Asia," *Human Vaccines and Immunotherapeutics* 18, no. 1 (2022), DOI: https://doi.org /10.1080/21645515.2021.2016010.
61 Ibid.
62 Ibid.
63 Ibid.
64 Darini Rajasingam- Senanayake, "Of Vaccine Geopolitics & Pfizer's Guinea Pigs: Covid-19 As 'Over the Horizon' War In Strategic Sri Lanka?," *Colombo Telegraph*, September 20, 2021, https://www.colombotelegraph.com/index. php/of-vaccine-geopolitics-pfizers-guinea-pigs-covid-19-as-over-the-horizon-war-in-strategic-sri-lanka/.
65 Ibid.
66 Sanjaya Lall and Senaka Bibile, "The Political Economy of Controlling Transnationals: The Pharmaceutical Industry in Sri Lanka (1972–76), *World Development* 5, no. 8 (1977): 677–97.
67 Nirmala Ganapathy, "India Losing Ground in its COVID-19 Vaccine Diplomacy Plan in South Asia," *The Straits Times*, June 3, 2021, https://www.straitstimes.com/asia/south-asia/india-losing-ground-in-its-south-asia-covid-19-vaccine-diplomacy-plan.
68 Alyson Bailes, Bradley Thyer and Baldur Thorhallson, "Alliance Theory and Alliance 'Shelter': The Complexities of Small State Alliance Behavior," *Third World Thematics: A TWQ Journal* 1, no. 1 (2016): 9–26. The concept of alliance "shelter" is based on five assumptions. First, small states not only differ in capabilities but are fundamentally different social units that operate in a different logic compared to their larger counterparts. Second, small states enter into alliance with larger states for domestic reasons as much as for international ones. Third, the lack of capabilities of small states allows them to benefit disproportionately from international cooperation in a manner denied to large states. Fourth, small states need political, economic and societal shelter as well as security protection to thrive. A common characteristic of small states is vulnerability to external factors such as reliance on foreign markets. Fifth, an alliance of shelter allows the small state to avoid isolation with the outside world by using their alliances.
69 Amit Ranjan, "The Maldives' Geopolitical Dilemma: India-China Rivalry, and Entry of the USA," *Asian Affairs* 52, no. 2 (2021): 375–95.
70 David Brewster, "Maldives: India First or India Out?," *The Interpreter*, November 24, 2021, https://www.lowyinstitute.org/the-interpreter/maldives-india-first-or-india-out.
71 Ranjan, "The Maldives' Geopolitical Dilemma," 380.
72 Press Release, "Bangladeshi Team to Join 'COVID Dhifaau' Campaign, Upon Request of the President," *The President's Office: Republic of the Maldives*, March 2, 2021, Reference No. 2021–048, https://presidency.gov.mv/Press/ Article/24391.
73 Vinitha Revi, "Sri Lanka and Maldives: Island Nations Look to China and Russia for Vaccines," in *The Dynamics of Vaccine Diplomacy in India's Neighbourhood*, Sohini Bose edited (New Delhi: Observer Research Foundation Report No. 145, 2021), https://www.orfonline.org/research/ the-dynamics-of-vaccine-diplomacy-in-indias-neighbourhood/.
74 ADB, "Republic of Maldives: Supporting COVID-19 Response and Vaccination Program," *Technical Assistance Project*, Project No. 55086–002, November 2021 (Manila: Asian Development Bank, 2021), https:// www.adb.org/sites/ default/files/project-documents/55086/55086-002-tar-en.pdf.

75 Ibid.
76 "India Starts Vaccine Shipments to Neighbours, Barring Pakistan and China," *Dawn*, January 20, 2021, https://www.dawn.com/news/1602575.
77 "Government Allots $1 Billion for Vaccine Procurement," *Dawn*, June 9, 2021, https://www.dawn.com/news/1628307.
78 Saaransh Mishra, "Pakistan and Afghanistan: Defining Equations in the Time of COVID-19," in *The Dynamics of Vaccine Diplomacy in India's Neighbourhood*, Sohini Bose edited (New Delhi: Observer Research Foundation Report No. 145, 2021), https://www.orfonline.org/research/the-dynamics-of-vaccine-diplomacy-in-indias-neighbourhood/.
79 Stuti Bhatnagar and Zahid Shahab Ahmed, "Geopolitics of Landlocked States in South Asia: A Comparative Analysis of Afghanistan and Nepal," *Australian Journal of International Affairs* (2020), DOI: 10.1080/10357718.2020.1793896.
80 Mishra, "Pakistan and Afghanistan."
81 The official statistics reveal a significant undercount. On the contrary, in a survey backed by the WHO, nearly ten million Afghans or nearly a third of the country's population was infected with COVID-19 as of 2020. See Ruchi Kumar, "Donated by India, Vaccines May Expire in Afghanistan," *Undark*, May 27, 2021, https://undark.org/2021/05/27/afghanistan-unused-vaccines-about-to-expire/.
82 Ibid.
83 Ibid.
84 See for e.g., Nigel Hawkes, "Doctor who Helped Locate bin Laden Worked for the CIA," *BMJ* 344 (2012): e785, DOI: 10.1136/bmj.e785.
85 Ruchi Kumar, "Donated by India."
86 See for e.g., Thomas Abraham, "What Has Gone Wrong with India's Vaccination Programme?," *The India Forum: A Journal-Magazine on Contemporary Issues* (April 16, 2021), https://www.theindiaforum.in/article/what-gone-wrong-india-s-vaccination-programme.
87 Jay Mazoomdar, "How Good Intentions but Bad Timing, Not Securing Stocks, Paved Road to the Shortage," *The Indian Express*, May 11, 2021, https://indianexpress.com/article/explained/covid-vaccination-vaccine-export-coronavirus-cases-7307604/.
88 "IISS Fullerton Lecture by S. Jaishankar, Foreign Secretary in Singapore," *Ministry of External Affairs Government of India Media Center*, July 20, 2015, https://mea.gov.in/Speeches-Statements.htm?dtl/25493/IISS_Fullerton_Lecture_by_Foreign_Secretary_in_Singapore.
89 Bhutta, Mitra, Salman et al., "Conflict, Extremism, Resilience and Peace in South Asia."
90 Ingrid Katz, Rebecca Weintraub, Linda Gail Bekker et al., "From Vaccine Nationalism to Vaccine Equity: Finding A Path Forward," *The New England Journal of Medicine* 384 (2021): 1281–83.
91 Thomas Bollyky and Chad Brown, "Vaccine Nationalism Will Prolong the Pandemic," *Foreign Affairs*, December 29, 2020, https://www.foreignaffairs.com/articles/world/2020-12-29/vaccine-nationalism-will-prolong-pandemic.
92 Shashika Bandara, Soumyadeep Bhoumik, Veena Sriram et al., "Stronger Together: A New Pandemic Agenda for South Asia," *BMJ Global Health* 6 (2021): e006776, DOI: http://dx.doi.org/10.1136/bmjgh-2021-006776.
93 Sophie Herman, Parsa Erfani, Tinashe Gorogna et al., "Global Vaccine Equity Demands Reparative Justice—Not Charity," *BMJ Global Health* 6 (2021): e0006504, DOI: 10.1136/bmjgh-2021-006504.
94 Ibid.
95 Bandara, Bhoumik, Sriram et al., "Stronger Together."

Index

Addu Atoll 79, 82, 84, 85, 91, 92
Afghanistan: conspiracy theories 151;
    COVID-19, response to 18;
    COVID-19 vaccine and CIA inter-
    ference, claims regarding 151;
    Hepatitis-B vaccination campaign
    151; malaria demonstration project
    36; National Malaria Organization
    and typhus control 38; SAARC
    membership 4; and transfer of mem-
    bership from SEARO to EMRO 34;
    vaccine skepticism and hesitancy 151
AFRO (WHO African Regional
    Office) 10
AIIHPH (All India Institute of Hygiene
    and Public Health) 57
AIIMS (All India Institute of Medical
    Sciences) 54, 57, 58, 64, 65
alliance of shelter 149
Alma Ata Declaration on Primary
    Healthcare: and Cold War misunder-
    standings 13; health, definition of 14
ambulatory chemoprophylaxis 40
ancylostomiasis 38
Anutin Chanvirakul 112
APSED (Asia Pacific Strategy on
    Emerging Infectious Diseases) 6, 121
ASA (Association of Southeast Asia) 4
ASEAN (Association of Southeast
    Asian Nations): ASEAN COVID-19
    Response Fund 19; ASEAN
    Free Trade Area 5; ASEAN
    Risk Assessment and Risk
    Communication Center 19; ASEAN
    Way 121; establishment of 120–21;
    health and regional integration,
    identification of 5; multilateral
    response to the pandemic 133;
    principle of non-interference 133

ASEAN Way 121
Asia Foundation 18, 99, 133
Asian-African Conference 11, 15, 16,
    42, 65, 66.
Asian-African Conference,
    Communiqué 11, 12, 15, 16, 42
Asian Development Bank 7, 149
Asian Financial Crisis 121
Associate Member: definition 34; and
    France, Pondicherry; Netherlands
    and inclusion in SEARO, compli-
    cations 34; and Portugal, Goa and
    Daman and Diu, representation
    of 34; Third WHA 34; and USSR
    SEARO membership proposal,
    withdrawal from 34–35; and UK,
    Maldives representation of 34
Atma Nirbhar Bharat (self-Sufficient
    India) 145, 151

Bandung Conference *see* Asian-African
    Conference
Bandung Plan 41, 98
Bandung Spirit: non-aligned foreign
    policy 45; and self-sufficiency in
    economic affairs 15; and Third-
    Worldism 12
Bangladesh: and Belt and Road initia-
    tive 146; coronavirus vaccine clinical
    trials, Sinovac Biotech controversy
    146; nationwide COVID-19
    lockdown 152
Barisan Nasional (National Front)
    Malaysia 127
BBIN (Bangladesh, Bhutan, India,
    Nepal) 22n9
BCG campaign: SEARO, assistance
    from 36; UNICEF, support from 39;
    and India, resistance from 39